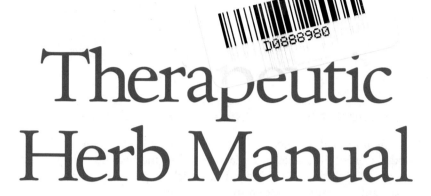

Therapeutic Herb Manual

A Guide to the Safe and Effective Use of Liquid Herbal Extracts

BY ED SMITH

"To take medicine only when you are sick is like digging a
well only when you are thirsty. Is it not already too late?"

Ch'i Po, circa 2500 BC

This manual is for educational and research purposes only.

It is not intended to medically prescribe or promote the sale of any product, nor is it intended to replace qualified medical healthcare. If you have, or think you have a condition which requires medical attention, you should promptly seek qualified healthcare.

Published by:
Ed Smith
P.O. Box 116
Williams, Oregon 97544

Printed in Oregon using recycled paper.

ACKNOWLEDGMENT

A special thanks to Richo Cech for his research assistance, and to Sara Katz and Tanya Guzman for their help in preparing this book for publication and their patience with me during the process.

PREFACE

The purpose of this book is to serve as a "ready reference" on the safe and effective use of liquid herbal extracts, and is by no means a definitive work on the herbs included. Although much of the language used throughout this text is in the vernacular of modern orthodox medicine, and diseases are often referred to by specific medical names, it must be understood that in traditional herbal medicine disease is not seen as a separate entity and therefore is not treated as such. Disease is actually an interrelated set of underlying conditions manifesting as a specific set of symptoms. Modern medical science classifies these symptoms into collective categories, gives each category a name (e.g., eczema, cancer, hypertension, etc.), and then tries to cure the patient by treating the symptoms. The herbalist, however, is more concerned with treating the patient, not the disease, and does so by improving the overall health of the patient and by removing the underlying causes of the disease.

Herbs by themselves can only be expected to do so much. For optimal results they should be used in the context of a natural wholesome diet, ample exercise and rest, a positive attitude, fulfilling work, and a simple lifestyle. This combination will almost always have a favorable influence on one's health and often induces healing where modern medicine has failed. The information presented in the following pages has been gleaned from 25 years of experience as a medical herbalist and from extensive academic research of herbal literature that range from ancient herbal texts to modern phytopharmaceutical journals. However, it must be understood that there can never be any guarantees that herbs will always help or heal every health problem for which they are indicated. There is no form of medicine, herbal or otherwise, that can make such a guarantee.

The Price of Freedom is Responsibility

It is every American's inherent right to freely choose for themselves whatever type and source of healthcare he or she deems appropriate. However, it must be emphasized that practicing such medical freedom requires the responsibility of acquiring valid health information and skills, having the wisdom to recognize when professional healthcare is needed, and to choose that healthcare wisely.

TABLE OF CONTENTS

HERBAL COMPOUNDS

SINGLE
HERB
EXTRACTS

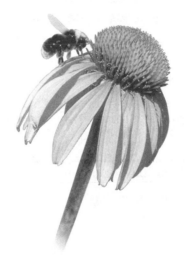

ALFALFA
Medicago sativa

Liquid extract of the spray-dried juice of whole herb.

Actions : Nourishing tonic that promotes appetite and weight gain. Galactogogue.

Uses: Indicated in anemia, poor appetite and wasting diseases. A tonic for nursing mothers.

Dose: Take 30 to 40 drops, 3 to 5 times per day.

Cautions: None known.

ANGELICA
Angelica archangelica

Liquid extract of dried first-year root.

Actions: Aromatic, digestion-enhancing bitters. Carminative. Diaphoretic. Anti-inflammatory.

Uses: Poor digestion and loss of appetite; flatulence; fever, colds and coughs; menstrual cramps; asthma; arthritis and rheumatism. When taken with hot water it gives warming relief from chills and coldness.

Dose: Take 30 to 40 drops, 2 to 5 times per day. To enhance appetite and digestion take 15 minutes before meals.

Cautions: Avoid large doses during pregnancy.

ANISE
Pimpinella anisum

Liquid extract of dried mature seed.

Actions: Pleasant tasting aromatic that is an excellent carminative, expectorant, and flavorful corrigent. Galactagogue.

Uses: Flatulence, indigestion and infant colic; hiccough. Coughs and bronchial catarrh.

Dose: Take 30 to 40 drops, 2 to 5 times per day.

Cautions: Avoid large doses during pregnancy.

ARNICA
Arnica montana
Liquid extract of dried flowers (1:10 herb/extract ratio).

Actions: Anti-inflammatory and resolvent actions promote dissipation and absorption of tissues destroyed by traumatic injury or over-exertion. Increases nerve force.

Uses: Traumatic injury, bruises, and sore strained joints, muscles, ligaments and tendons; tensive backache; concussion; stroke; heart strain and debility of heart muscle due to over-excitement or over-activity; post-partum discomfort and muscular soreness; reduces pain and bleeding during and after surgery and facilates recovery. Emotional trauma (e.g., sudden bad news, terror, violence). Sadness and depression. Poor blood circulation, and urinary incontinence due to weak nerve force. Topically apply over strained sore areas, and insect bites and stings. Gargle for sore throat or laryngitis.

Dose: Take 5 to 10 drops in full cup of water, 1 to 3 times per day. Best given in small, well-diluted doses (These doses are based on the 1:10 extract only.) Topically apply cotton cloth wetted with mixture of 1 teaspoon extract and a cup of cool water. Renew every 1 or 2 hours. As gargle mix 5 to 10 drops in half-cup water and gargle several times per day.

Cautions: Avoid or moderate use in excitment of the nervous system, irritation of stomach and intestines, acute inflammation, high fever or asthma. Excessive doses can cause nervous excitement and throat and stomach irritation. Prolonged topical use, or application to broken skin may cause skin irritation. Discontinue use if these symptoms appear.

ASHWAGANDHA
Withania somnifera
Liquid extract of dry root.

Actions: Adaptogenic tonic that promotes vitality and vigor. Sexual tonic. Nervine sedative.

Uses: Tiredness and general debility; nervous and sexual debility; lack of concentration and memory loss; drug burnout. Headache.

Dose: Take 30 to 40 drops, 2 or 3 times per day. Often taken with milk in traditional Ayurvedic medicine.

Cautions: Moderate use during pregnancy.

ASTRAGALUS
Astragalus membranaceus
Liquid extract of dried root (extracted with heat).

Actions: Nourishes vital force ("chi"). General immune system tonic; increases production and activity of undifferentiated immune cells, and interferon. Builds blood. Promotes endurance and stamina. Liver protective and restorative.

Uses: As convalescence tonic in general debility and weakness. Weak immune system and wasting illness; protective of immune cells during chemo or radiation treatments; prevent or moderate colds and flu. Strengthening lung tonic; soothes coughs. Poor appetite. Anemia. Chronic liver maladies.

Dose: Take 30 to 40 drops, 3 or 4 times per day.

Cautions: Avoid or moderate use with acute inflammation or fever.

BASIL
Ocimum basilicum
Liquid extract of fresh leaf.

Actions: Soothing to stomach. Mildly sedative. Soothing expectorant. Diaphoretic. Aromatic, flavorful corrigent.

Uses: Nausea; morning sickness or motion sickness. Flatulence. Nervousness. Thick coughs. Withdrawal from marijuana addiction.

Dose: Take 30 to 40 drops, 3 to 5 times per day.

Cautions: None known.

BAYBERRY
Myrica cerifera
Liquid extract of dried root bark (no adhering wood).

Actions: Stimulating, warming astringent.

Uses: Atonic, sluggish mucous membranes and excessive mucous discharge; atonic leucorrhea; chronic catarrh of sinuses, stomach and intestines, and the urinary tract; stomach and intestinal ulcers; gargle or rinse for sore throat, mouth sores and bleeding, spongy gums.

Dose: Take 30 to 40 drops, 2 to 4 times per day. As gargle mix drops in a little water and gargle several times per day.

Cautions: Avoid or moderate use in acute inflammatory conditions and fever.

BLACK COHOSH
Cimicifuga racemosa
Liquid extract of dried rhizome & rootlets.

Actions: Antispasmodic and antirheumatic. Isoflavones ("phytoestrogens") bind to estrogen receptors and have mild estrogen-like activity. Promotes effectual labor contractions, relieves false labor pains, and facilitates post-partum recovery.

Uses: Dull, aching, contractive muscle pains (esp. rheumatic and myalgic pains). Low-estrogen conditions. Premenstrual syndrome (PMS); painful, weak, irregular or delayed menstruation. Menopause. Weak, irregular labor contractions; relief of false labor pains; post-partum uterine soreness.

Dose: Take 30 to 40 drops, 2 to 4 times per day. During labor take 30 to 40 drops in hot water every 20 to 30 minutes if needed.

Cautions: During pregnancy or labor use only under direction of a qualified midwife. Excessive dosage can cause nausea, light headedness and dull headache.

BLADDERWRACK
Fucus vesiculosus & *F. distichus*
Liquid extract of dried fertile thallus.

Actions: Nutritive alterative. Contains significant levels of dietary iodine.

Uses: Under-active thyroid and associated sluggish metabolism, obesity, atonic uterine tissues and menstrual irregularity; tonic for torpid persons, with cold, clammy skin. Relieves irritation and chronic inflammation of bladder.

Dose: Take 30 to 40 drops, 2 to 4 times per day.

Cautions: Avoid or moderate use in hyperthyroid (over-active thyroid gland).

BLESSED THISTLE
Cnicus benedictus
Liquid extract of dried flowering herb.

Actions: Digestive bitter that tonifies stomach. Taken hot is diaphoretic and promotes menstrual flow. Galactagogue.

Uses: Loss of appetite, atonic dyspepsia and poor digestion (esp. fats); sluggish liver. Suppressed menses due to colds or chill. Beginning of fevers and inflammations.

Dose: Take 30 to 40 drops, 2 to 4 times per day. To enhance appetite and digestion take 15 minutes before meals.

Cautions: High doses may cause nausea.

BLOODROOT
Sanguinaria canadensis
Liquid extract of dried rhizome.

Actions: Stimulates mucous membrane secretions; expectorant. Topical antifungal.

Uses: Sluggish mucous membranes; general atonic conditions of sinuses, lungs and bronchi, (esp. in harsh, dry coughs). Sluggish capillary circulation of skin, and cold extremities. Topically against ringworm or warts.

Dose: Take 10 to 20 drops in half-cup of water, 2 to 4 times per day. Topically, wet wart or fungus area several times a day, but avoid applying to surrounding healthy areas.

Cautions: Do not take extract undiluted. Lower dosage or discontinue use if stomach irritation, nausea, vomiting or other distressful symptoms occur. Do not take during pregnancy or nursing.

BLUE COHOSH
Caulophyllum thalictroides
Liquid extract of dried rhizome & roots.

Actions: Antispasmodic and antirheumatic. Uterine tonic. Promotes effectual labor contractions, and averts premature labor; facilitates post-partum recovery.

Uses: Threatened miscarriage. Menstrual cramps and discomfort (esp. "heavy legs"); excessive flow. Menopause pains and discomfort. Weak and irritable nervous system; nervous insomnia.

Dose: Take 30 to 40 drops, 3 to 4 times per day.

Cautions: For use during pregnancy or labor consult qualified midwife.

BLUE FLAG

Iris versicolor

Liquid extract of fresh rhizome & roots.

Actions: Alterative, cholagogue and laxative in moderate doses, and emetic and cathartic in large doses. Increases secretions of salivary glands, liver, gallbladder, pancreas, spleen and intestines. Promotes excretion of metabolic wastes, and corrects faulty, retrograde metabolism and associated blood, lymphatic and glandular toxicity.

Uses: Wasting diseases associated with chronic, torpid conditions: non-malignant enlargement of spleen, thyroid (esp. with menstrual, ovarian and uterine disorders), and lymphatics (soft and yielding lymph nodes); enlarged uterus or ovaries, leukorrhea, congestive dysmenorrhea, ulceration of os and cervix, and uterine fibroids. Rheumatic conditions. Liver and gall bladder torpor and congestion due to venous and lymphatic stasis; jaundice, chronic hepatitis and other chronic liver disorders, with flatulence, constipation or clay-colored stools; headache, vertigo, nausea or vomiting caused by indigestion or biliousness, especially after eating fats. Alterative in various skin conditions, especially if skin is inactive, jaundiced, or is rough and greasy. Indicated in pustular eruptions, acne and disorders of the sebaceous glands; ulcerating or oozing skin diseases; chronic and persistent psoriasis or eczema.

Dose: For normal, gentle action, extract is best taken in small doses, well diluted, and repeated at short intervals. Mix 40 to 60 drops into half-cup water and take 1 teaspoon every 1 or 2 hours (mix well before each dose).

For stronger, more pronounced action mix 10 to 20 drops into half-cup water and drink all at once -- do this 2 or 3 times per day. These stronger doses are best combined with demulcents (e.g., Marshmallow or Comfrey) and carminatives (e.g., Fennel or Anise).

For most adults, maximum total dose should not exceed 60 drops per 24-hour-period, or even less for more sensitive individuals, and should not be taken for longer than 1 week.

Cautions: Do not take extract undiluted. Lower dosage or discontinue use if abdominal pain, nausea, vomiting, diarrhea or other distressful symptoms occur. Avoid, or take in very small, well diluted doses, during pregnancy or breast feeding, and in fever and acute inflammatory conditions.

BONESET
Eupatorium perfoliatum
Liquid extract of dried leaf & flowering tops.

Actions: Gently laxative. Diaphoretic. Promotes and enhances immune system function.

Uses: Poor appetite and digestion. Fevers; cold or flu, especially with chills and deep-seated muscle ache ("achey bones"); chronic coughs and bronchitis; pneumonia. Poor immune response and slow recovery.

Dose: Take 30 to 40 drops, 3 to 5 times per day. Take in hot water with Ginger for colds, flu and chills.

Cautions: Large doses may cause nausea.

BUCHU
Agothosma betulina
Liquid extract of dried leaf.

Actions: Stimulant, antiseptic, cleansing and tonic to the kidneys, bladder and mucous membranes of the urinary tract. Mild diuretic action increases elimination of both watery and solid constituents of urine. However, it moderates excessive activity of kidneys.

Uses: Chronic, atonic diseases of the urinary system, or chronic irritation with discharge (especially in the aged). Abnormally acid or muddy urine loaded with salts, with constant desire to urinate but with little relief from the effort. Chronic cystitis, urethritis, prostatitis, gonorrhea, pyuria (pus in urine) and gleet. Incontinence associated with prostate maladies.

Dose: Take 30 to 60 drops in half-cup water, 2 to 4 times per day.

Cautions: Do not use in acute inflammations of urinary tract. Sensitive individuals may experience gastrointestinal intolerance; avoid taking on an empty stomach. Moderate use during pregnancy. Buchu can harmlessly impart its aroma to the urine and render it dark in color.

BUGLEWEED
Lycopus americanus

Liquid extract of dried flowering herb.

Actions: Counteracts excess thyroxine (thyroid gland hormone). Circulatory and heart sedative; nervous system sedative. Hemostatic (allays minor bleeding).

Uses: Hyperthyroid (overactive thyroid gland). Heart problems marked by irritable, accelerated or irregular heart action (esp. with sense of oppression in chest with difficult breathing); reduces pulse and restores circulatory and cardiac tone. Coughs with copious expectoration (esp. chronic debilitating coughs). Mild bleeding of lungs, stomach, intestines, uterus or urinary tract. Insomnia.

Dose: Take 30 to 40 drops, 3 to 5 times per day.

Cautions: Thyroid enlargement or hypothyroid (underactive thyroid). Consult with physician before taking with thyroid drugs. Moderate use during pregnancy.

BURDOCK
Arctium lappa

Blended liquid extracts of dried root & mature seed.

Actions: Excellent blood and lymph purifier (alterative) that promotes elimination of metabolic waste (esp. to skin, mucous membranes and kidneys). Promotes and enhances immune system function. Soothing and cleansing diuretic. Supports immune system function.

Uses: Various skin maladies, including hives, psoriasis, eczema, acne and boils (esp. greasy skin). Ulcerations of skin and mucous membranes. Chronic glandular enlargements. Arthritis and gout. Irritation of bladder and urethra. Compromised or weak immune system.

Dose: Take 30 to 40 drops, 3 or 4 times per day.

Cautions: Excessive doses may cause aching in kidneys and lower back due to over-active cleansing. Lower dosage or discontinue use if this happens.

BUTCHER'S BROOM
Ruscus aculeatus
Liquid extract of dried rhizome.

Actions: Anti-inflammatory tonic for the veins. Reduces capillary fragility and permeability and tones sluggish venous system.

Uses: Extremities & skin: varicose veins, varicose ulcers and phlebitis, painful veins, leg edema and cramps (esp. during pregnancy); frostbite, chilblains, purpura, Raynaud's disease. Anorectum: reduces swelling, pain, heat and itching of hemorrhoids and anal fissures. Retina: diabetic retinopathy and retinal bleeding. Gynecological: vein disorders related to oral contraceptives, premenstrual syndrome (PMS), certain menstrual disorders. Post-operative: taken before and after surgery to prevent or minimize postoperative thrombosis (esp. where anticoagulant therapy is contraindicated).

Dose: Take 30 to 40 drops, 3 to 5 times per day. For compress, wet cloth with mixture of 1 teaspoonful of extract in half-cup water. Renew compress every 1 or 2 hours. Topical use is enhanced if extract is also taken internally.

Cautions: None known.

CACTUS (Cactus grandiflorus)
Selenicereus grandiflorus
Liquid extract of fresh flower & succulent stem.

Actions: Excellent heart and nerve tonic (contains no cardiac glycosides). Normalizes heart rhythm and strengthens contractile force.

Uses: Cardiac weakness (esp. with feeble irregular pulse). Nervous disorders with weak heart beat, poor circulation, mental depression and fear. Poor memory, and erectile dysfunction due to inadequate circulation. Nervous heart, hot flashes and general melancholy during menopause. Hypochondria with fear of death.

Dose: Take 30 to 40 drops, 2 or 3 times per day. Best results are seen when combined with Hawthorn and Avena, and taken for several months.

Cautions: Not reliable in emergency cardiac cases.

CALAMUS
Acorus calamus var. *Americanus*

Liquid extract of dried unpeeled rhizome.

Actions: Aromatic bitters and carminative that stimulates appetite and enhances good digestion. Tonic to mucous membranes of mouth and throat. Deters taste for tobacco. Sharpens memory.

Uses: Poor appetite, poor digestion and dyspepsia; pain and uneasiness in stomach and bowels; intestinal gas; diarrhea and dysentery. Coughs, bronchitis and chest colds. Tobacco addiction. Failing memory due to old age or drug abuse.

Dose: Take 30 to 40 drops, 2 to 4 times per day. To improve appetite and digestion take 15 minutes before meals.

Cautions: European and Asian varieties contain the potentially toxic compound, ß-asarone, which is not found in the North American variety, *Acorus calamus* var. *Americanus.*

CALENDULA
Calendula officinalis

Liquid extract of dried flowers.

Actions: Excellent vulnerary that promotes healing of skin; anti-inflammatory. Topical antibacterial and antiviral.

Uses: Cuts, abrasions and burns; bacterial infections of the skin; ulcerations and sores of the mouth, throat or skin; herpes; varicose veins and hemorrhoids; insect stings; bruises and "black eye."

Dose: Take 30 to 40 drops, 2 to 5 times per day. As a dressing or wash use full-strength (if well tolerated), or dilute with 2 to 3 parts water.

Cautions: None known.

CALIFORNIA POPPY
Eschscholzia californica

Liquid extract of fresh whole flowering plant with root.

Actions: Contains sedative alkaloids similar to the Opium Poppy alkaloids, yet are very safe and non-addictive. Antispasmodic, analgesic (quiets pain) and soporific (induces sleep).

Uses: Anxiety, restlessness and insomnia. Headache, toothache, and general neuropathies. Is tolerated well by children, and is especially indicated in bed-wetting associated with nervousness.

Dose: Take 30 to 40 drops, 2 to 5 times per day.

Cautions: Moderate use during pregnancy.

CARDAMON
Elettaria cardamomum
Liquid extract of dried, semi-mature capsule with seed (unbleached).

Actions: Warming stomachic and carminative. Gentle liver and bile stimulant. Diuretic. Delicious aromatic corrigent.

Uses: Flatulence and colic. Nausea and mild stomach disturbances. Agreeable addition to liver, gallbladder and digestive formulas. Flavoring for syrups, compounds, etc. (esp. bitters and laxatives).

Dose: Take 30 to 40 drops, 2 to 5 times per day.

Cautions: None known.

CATNIP
Nepeta cataria
Liquid extract of fresh leaf & flowering tops.

Actions: Mild sedative and antispasmodic . Mild carminative. Mild diaphoretic to lower fevers. Excellent remedy for children.

Uses: Indigestion, dyspepsia, flatulence and infant's colic. Fevers, colds and flu. Nervousness, restlessness, sleeplessness and nervous headache; persistent crying. Menstrual maladies accompanied by nervous tension.

Dose: Take 30 to 40 drops, 2 to 5 times per day in hot water.

Cautions: None known.

CAT'S CLAW (Uña de Gato)
Uncaria tomentosa
Liquid extract of dried inner bark (no adhering wood).

Actions: Promotes and enhances immune system function; antiviral. Antimutagenic; neutralizes tobbaco and other mutagens in the urine. Anti-inflammatory and antirheumatic. Antifertility action deters implanting of fertilized egg.

Uses: Rheumatism and arthritis. Gastritis and ulcers. As adjunct therapy in the treatment of cancer and other conditions associated with a compromised immune system. As protective therapy for tobacco smokers.

Dose: Take 30 to 40 drops, 3 to 5 times per day.

Cautions: May prevent conception. Although there is no evidence of abortative activity, use during pregnancy is cautioned.

CAYENNE
Capsicum annuum var. *frutescens*
Liquid extract of dried ripe peppers with seeds.

Actions: Simple but powerful warming stimulant to heart, blood circulation, nervous system and mucous membranes, but does not excite or quicken the pulse. Promotes action of secreting organs. Topical stimulant, rubefacient and analgesic.

Uses: Poor circulation, cold extremities and pallid face. Weak nerve force. Torpid digestive system with indigestion and flatulence. Repressed secretions and to expel thick mucous. Hoarseness. Fevers. Alcoholic delirium tremens; opium and heroin addiction. Topically applied for rheumatic joint pain; nerve pain; shingles.

Dose: Take 10 to 30 drops, 2 to 5 times per day in half-cup water. Topically apply full-strength (if well tolerated), or dilute with 2 or 3 parts rubbing alcohol.

Cautions: Do not take drops undiluted. Excessive internal doses may cause stomach irritation. Counteract with demulcent or fatty drinks (e.g., Marshmallow root, Slippery Elm bark or milk). Avoid contact with broken skin, eyes and mucous membranes. If topical use causes painful heating, wash area with hot soapy water or rubbing alcohol; flush eyes with lots of cool water.

CELANDINE
Chelidonium majus
Liquid extract of fresh whole flowering plant with root.

Actions: Stimulates liver and gallbladder secretions and drainage (cholagogue); antispasmodic to gallbladder and gastrointestinal tract. Removes warts.

Uses: Inefficient function of glandular organs of abdominal cavity, and sluggish and deficient circulation of tissues, glands and organs of this cavity; inflammation and congestion of liver, gallbladder and spleen; liver related headaches and dyspepsia; diminished bile secretion and relief of gallbladder congestion; prevention of gallstone colic; gastrointestinal spasms. Topically for removal of warts and corns.

Dose: Take 30 to 40 drops, 2 or 3 times per day in half-cup of water. Apply full-strength to warts or corns 3 or 4 times per day.

Cautions: Moderate use during pregnancy. Larger doses may cause nausea or diarrhea.

CELERY
Apium graveolens
Blended liquid extracts of dried whole plant with root, & mature seed.

Actions: Restorative nerve tonic and sedative. Mild diuretic and urinary antiseptic. Antirheumatic. Digestive tonic.

Uses: Arthritis, rheumatism and gout. Indigestion and flatulence. Urinary tract inflammation and infection. Neurasthenia (nervous depletion); and sleeplessness; anxiety and nervous breakdown.

Dose: Take 30 to 40 drops, 2 to 5 times per day.

Cautions: Moderate use during pregnancy.

CHAMOMILE
Matricaria chamomilla
Liquid extract of fresh flowers.

Actions: Antispasmodic and calming sedative. Digestant, stomachic and carminative. Anti-inflammatory and vulnerary. Diaphoretic. Excellent remedy for children.

Uses: Nervous irritability (esp. in children and the aged); nervous, peevish children (esp. during teething); nervousness during pregnancy, and false pains; premenstrual syndrome (PMS) and nervousness during menses; delayed menses due to chill or nervousness; nervous cough; nervous stomach and intestinal cramps; flatulence and colic. Inflammatory conditions (esp. gastrointestinal); gastric or intestinal ulcers; nervous diarrhea. Bedwetting caused by bladder irritation. Fevers, colds and flu.

Dose: Take 30 to 40 drops, 2 to 5 times per day. Take in hot water to promote sweating and abate colds.

Cautions: None known.

CHASTE TREE
Vitex agnus-castus
Liquid extract of dried mature berry.

Actions: Enhances natural production of progesterone and luteinizing hormone, and diminishes release of follical stimulating hormone.

Uses: Menstrual and ovulation disorders due to corpus luteum insufficiency: amenorrhea, hypermenorrhea and polymenorrhea; excess prolactin levels; to induce ovulation in infertility; premenstrual syndrome (PMS); breast pain; normalize ovulation and menstrual cycle after quitting oral contraceptives. Cysts and fibroids of the breasts, ovaries and uterus. Menopausal depression and hypochondria. Galactagogue (promotes breast milk). Decreases abnormally strong libido in men.

Dose: Take 30 to 40 drops, 2 or 3 times per day.

Cautions: Discontinue or lower dosage if extract causes nausea, diarrhea or abnormal changes in menstrual cycle. Moderate use during pregnancy.

CLEAVERS
Galium aparine
Liquid extract of dried whole herb
harvested as flowers are just emerging.

Actions: Soothing diuretic. Lymphatic and glandular alterative which facilitates removal of catabolic wastes and facilitates repair of tissue. Cooling to fevers (but is not diaphoretic).

Uses: Irritation or inflammation of urinary tract; dysuria and painful urination; to clear urinary wastes and mucous. Lymphatic and glandular swellings. Ovarian cysts. Benign prostatic hypertrophy (BPH) and other prostate maladies. Psoriasis, eczema, hives and skin problems associated with poor elimination (esp. nodular deposits). Mononucleosis. Measles. Fevers.

Dose: Take 30 to 40 drops, 2 to 5 times per day.

Cautions: Avoid or combine with warming herbs when body is cold.

COLTSFOOT
Tussilago farfara
Liquid extract of fresh flowering tops (pyrrolizidine alkaloids removed).

Actions: Sedative to coughs; demulcent expectorant that thins and expels mucous in respiratory tract. Anti-inflammatory.

Uses: Coughs; infection of upper respiratory tract, with thick mucous and cough; asthma, bronchitis, hoarseness, laryngitis.

Dose: Take 30 to 40 drops, 2 to 5 times per day.

Cautions: Avoid Coltsfoot preparations containing pyrrolizidine alkaloids.

COMFREY
Symphytum officinale
Liquid extract of fresh root (pyrrolizidine alkaloids removed).

Actions: Superb wound healer and cell-proliferant (vulnerary); anti-inflammatory. Demulcent and mildly astringent; expectorant.

Uses: Used internally and topically to heal cuts, abrasions, burns, ulcerations, bruises, broken bones, and strained ligaments and tendons (use internally and topically). Chronic inflammation, passive bleeding and excessive mucous discharge of gastrointestinal, urinary and respiratory tracts. Gastric and duodenal ulcers; colitis. Coughs (esp. dry unproductive type).

Dose: Take 30 to 60 drops, 2 to 5 times per day. Topically apply full-strength (if well tolerated), or dilute with 2 or 3 parts water.

Cautions: Avoid Comfrey preparations containing pyrrolizidine alkaloids. Take care on deep cuts or puncture wounds not to heal top of wound before inside of wound.

COPTIS
Chinese Goldthread & Huang Lian
Coptis chinensis
Liquid extract of dried rhizome.

Actions: Clears heat and dampness. Astringent. Anti-inflammatory. Antibacterial, antiviral and antiprotozoal. Cholagogue. Removes toxins and wastes from blood.

Uses: Infections and fevers, especially bacterial dysentery, hepatitis, respiratory infections, typhoid fever, and trichomal vaginitis (as douche). Astringent to ulcerations associated with gastroenteritis (inflammation of stomach and intestines) and colitis. Hemostatic for nosebleed and blood in urine, stool, sputum and vomit. Blood purifier for septicemia, carbuncles and abscesses, eruptive dermatitis and eczema. Chronic inflammation of stomach and intestines, and associated bad breath and putrid belching. Topically used as astringent disinfectant to wound, infections, ulcerations, skin eruptions, and ulcerations of mouth and throat (rinse or gargle).

Dose: Take 30 to 40 drops, 3 to 5 times per day. In acute fevers and infections 50 to 70 drops per dose can be taken for no more than 3 days. Topically apply full-strength (if well tolerated), or dilute with 2 or 3 parts water. As gargle mix drops in a little water and gargle several times per day.

Cautions: Moderate use during pregnancy.

CORN SILK
Zea mays
Liquid extract of fresh stigma & style ("silk") of corn ears.

Actions: Nutritive. Soothing diuretic. Mild heart and blood vessel tonic.

Uses: Irritations and inflammation of urinary tract (esp. alkaline urine); especially useful in children's bladder disorders and bedwetting due to irritation. Water retention caused by heart or kidney conditions.

Dose: Take 30 to 40 drops, 2 to 5 times per day.

Cautions: None known.

CRAMP BARK
Viburnum opulus
Liquid extract of dried, spring-harvested bark.

Actions: Balances symphathetic and parasympathetic nervous systems. Antispasmodic to tubular organs (i.e., stomach, intestines, uterus and bladder). Uterine and pregnancy tonic.

Uses: Menstrual cramps and nausea; sudden or irregular menstrual flow due to fevers. Painful spasms of uterus and ovaries with pain in thighs and back. Spastic pains during pregnancy; spotting, threatened miscarriage or false labor pains; post-partum pain and cramps. Leg cramps (esp. during pregnancy). Bladder stricture. To facilitate insertion of catheters.

Dose: Take 30 to 40 drops, 2 to 5 times per day.

Cautions: None known.

CULVER'S ROOT
Leptandra virginica
Liquid extract of dried rhizome & roots
(aged 1 year before extraction).

Actions: Mildly stimulates liver function, promotes secretion of bile, and removes accumulated detritus from the gall bladder. Gentle-acting laxative which stimulates peristalsis and cleanses digestive tract of viscid mucous. Improves digestive function. Gentle action especially indicated for children and the elderly.

Uses: Atony of liver, gallbladder and intestines, and enfeebled portal circulation; hepatitis, cholecystitis, and non-obstructive jaundice. Chronic constipation associated with liver congestion. Specific in chronic enteritis. Poor digestion and dyspepsia due to atony of the stomach and liver.

Dose: Take 30 to 40 drops, 2 to 4 times per day.

Cautions: Avoid large doses during pregnancy. Discontinue or lower dosage if extract causes abdominal pain.

DAMIANA
Turnera aphrodisiaca
Liquid extract of dried leaf & flower (minimal stem).

Actions: Flavorful aromatic. Mild sedative. Soothing tonic to sexual and urinary organs; purported to increase libido. Promotes healthy menstruation. Soothing diuretic and expectorant.

Uses: Nervous debility, anxiety and depression. Sexual atony or anxiety in men and women. Inflammation of sexual organs and urinary tract Menstrual maladies; taken hot it promotes tardy period (not abortive). Menopause. Respiratory irritation, coughs and hypersecretion.

Dose: Take 30 to 40 drops, 3 to 5 times per day.

Cautions: None known.

DANDELION
Taraxacum officinale
Liquid extract of fresh whole flowering plant with root.

Actions: Alterative. General tonic to digestive organs; improves appetite and digestion. Mild-acting cleanser and decongestant to liver and gallbladder; enhances bile flow; promotes regularity of bowel movements. Diuretic and kidney cleanser.

Uses: Retrograde metabolism. Liver congestion, bile duct obstruction or deficient bile secretion. Chronic dyspepsia and indigestion. Chronic constipation. Many maladies associated with liver derangements can benefit from Dandelion (esp. arthritis, gout and skin disorders).

Dose: Take 30 to 40 drops, 2 to 4 times per day. Best results are seen after several weeks of use.

Cautions: Liver cleansing can sometimes cause adverse reactions like nausea or colic (esp. with toxic liver or bile duct blockage). Lower dosage or discontinue use if this happens.

DEVIL'S CLAW
Harpagophytum procumbens
Liquid extract of dried, secondary tuber (not root).

Actions: Anti-inflammatory, antirheumatic and analgesic. Promotes appetite and digestion (esp. fats). Metabolic cleanser/detoxifier of blood, lymph, pancreas, liver and kidneys.

Uses: Arthritis and rheumatic problems; tendinitis; lower back pain. Poor appetite. Slow metabolism. Insufficient production of bile and related problems of digestion. Acne, psoriasis and other skin problems.

Dose: Take 30 to 40 drops, 2 to 4 times per day.

Cautions: Use in moderate doses with congested gallbladder or gallstones; larger doses may work too strongly and cause colic.

DEVIL'S CLUB
Oplopanax horridum
Liquid extract of dried root bark (no adhering wood)

Actions: Alterative, rejuvenating tonic that enhances physical endurance, stamina and overall good health, and optimizes longevity. In larger doses acts as a mild laxative.

Uses: Arthritis and rheumatism; fevers, colds, flu and coughs; hangover; stomach ailments; swollen glands; measles. Regulate menses after childbirth. Popular as Native American folk remedy for the control of diabetes.

Dose: Take 30 to 40 drops, 3 to 5 times per day.

Cautions: Do not change medical treatment of diabetes (esp. insulin dosage) without the advice of a qualified physician. Diabetics should monitor their blood sugar level and insulin needs carefully while taking Devil's Club.

ECHINACEA
Echinacea purpurea
Blended liquid extracts of fresh whole root,
fresh leaf & flower (no stem), & dried mature seed.

Actions: Immune system modulator and tonic. Anti-inflammatory. Stimulates healthy growth of connective tissue and speeds healing of damaged tissues. Excellent alterative, and blood and lymphatic cleanser.

Uses: All conditions where immune system is challenged or compromised: Inflammations, infections, fevers, colds, flu, allergies, etc. Weak immune system and susceptibility to infections or slow-healing wounds. Septicemia ("blood poisoning"). Lymphatic congestion. Boils and carbuncles. Eczema, psoriasis, hives and other skin problems. General "run-down" feeling. Arthritis. Venomous stings and bites.

Dose: Take 30 to 40 drops, 2 to 5 times per day. In fevers, severe infections, or venomous bites and stings doses can be as large as 40 to 80 drops every 1 to 2 hours (depending upon severity). As fever or symptoms subside, dosage can be lowered in size and frequency. Topically apply full strength (if well tolerated), or dilute with 1 or 2 parts water.

Cautions: Some say Echinacea is contraindicated in autoimmune diseases, and that long-continued doses cause therapeutic effects to diminish. However, there has been no scientific or clinical evidence of this, and traditional use of Echinacea demonstrates otherwise.

ELDER FLOWER
Sambucus canadensis
Liquid extract of dried flowering umbels.

Actions: Diaphoretic which helps lower fevers. Diuretic. Alterative that increases excretion and elimination of metabolic wastes.

Uses: Simple fevers, colds and flu. Bronchitis and to clear bronchial phlegm. Defective excretion and elimination; adema. Skin maladies caused by metabolic toxins, especially those with watery discharge like "weeping eczema" and dermatitis caused by poison ivy or poison oak.

Dose: Take 30 to 40 drops, 2 to 5 times per day. To induce sweat take 40 to 80 drops with hot water or tea and soak body in hot water. Topically apply full strength (if well tolerated) or dilute with 1 or 2 parts water.

Cautions: None known.

ELECAMPANE
Inula helenium
Liquid extract of dried second-year roots.

Actions: Stimulating, cleansing and tonic to mucous membranes. Excellent antiseptic expectorant. Alterative.

Uses: All affections of mucous membranes with excessive mucous secretions. Bronchial and lung irritation with teasing cough and abundant discharge; humid asthma; bronchitis; pneumonia; tuberculosis of lungs; other respiratory infections. Chronic mucous discharge from urinary bladder and the reproductive organs; leucorrhea; gleet. To cleanse stomach and intestines of excess mucous coating. Night sweats.

Dose: Take 30 to 40 drops, 2 to 5 times per day.

Cautions: Moderate use during pregnancy or nursing. Elecampane is best suited for wet coughs and not dry or unproductive coughs.

EYEBRIGHT
Euphrasia officinalis
Liquid extract of fresh flowering herb

Actions: Anti-inflammatory (and antihistamine) to mucous membranes of the eyes, ears, nose, sinuses, throat and bronchi.

Uses: Coughs, hoarseness, headache, conjunctivitis ("pink eye"), earache and sinusitis, especially when associated with watery mucous secretions with heat and pain; hayfever and other allergies; bronchitis. During or following measles to control inflammatory mucous discharge.

Dose: Take 30 to 40 drops, 2 to 5 times per day.

Cautions: None known.

FENNEL
Foeniculum vulgare
Liquid extract of dried mature seed.

Actions: Stomachic and carminative. Expectorant. Gentle liver and bile stimulant. Enhances production of breast milk. Aromatic flavoring and corrigent. Excellent remedy for children.

Uses: Indigestion, flatulence and fullness after meals; nausea and stomach disturbances; infant colic. Coughs and colds. Agreeable addition to liver, gallbladder and digestive formulas. Suppressed or insufficient lactation. Flavoring for syrups, compounds, etc. (esp. bitters and laxatives).

Dose: Take 30 to 40 drops, 2 to 5 times per day.

Cautions: None known.

FEVERFEW
Tanacetum parthenium
Liquid extract of dried leaf & flower.

Actions: Aspirin-like action relieves pain and reduces fever.

Uses: Headaches (esp. migraine) arthritis; fevers; menstrual cramps and pains; stomach ache; toothache.

Dose: Take 30 to 40 drops, 2 to 4 times per day.

Cautions: Rarely some sensitive individuals may have an allergic reaction to Feverfew. Discontinue use if this happens.

FRINGE TREE
Chionanthus virginicus
Liquid extract of dried root bark (no adhering wood).

Actions: Stimulates bile flow (cholagogue) and promotes liver action and drainage.

Uses: Hepatitis with enlarged liver; liver congestion and jaundice; clay-colored stools; alcoholic liver. Thins bile and deters formation of gallstones. Faulty digestion of fats. Excessive mucous discharge in stomach, gallbladder and intestines. Especially indicated by yellow skin and liver pain. Chronic inflammation of spleen, pancreas and kidneys.

Dose: Take 30 to 40 drops in a cup of water, 2 to 4 times per day.

Cautions: Use with caution in blockage of gallbladder; here combine with Wild Yam and/or Khella.

GARLIC
Allium sativum
Liquid extract of fresh whole bulb.

Actions: Antiseptic (antibacterial and antifungal). Metabolic stimulant. Clears phlegm; expectorant. Reduces cholesterol. Inhibits platelet aggregation ("thins the blood").

Uses: Heart disease associated with high cholesterol, fatty deposits and arteriosclerosis; high blood pressure. Infections of eyes, ears and throat; respiratory infections, coughs and hoarseness; colds and flu. Obesity.

Dose: Take 30 to 40 drops, 2 to 3 times per day. Mix with 20 drops of Peppermint Spirits to moderate Garlic odor.

Cautions: Discontinue, lower dosage or combine with Peppermint Spirits if digestive upset occurs. Avoid use in cases of inflamed stomach. May impart taste or odor of garlic to breast milk.

GINGER
Zingiber officinale
Liquid extract of dried rhizome.

Actions: Warming, aromatic flavor. Heart tonic and warming circulatory and metabolic stimulant. Stomachic, digestive and carminative; prevents or relieves nausea. Antispasmodic. Expectorant.

Uses: Atonic dyspepsia; pain and cramps of stomach and bowels; relieve stomach and intestinal gas. Diarrhea and dysentery. Nausea (esp. motion sickness). Fevers, colds and coughs. Cold skin, hands and feet. Painful menstruation. Heart disease and poor circulation. Hypercholesterol.

Dose: Take 30 to 40 drops in half-cup water, 2 to 5 times per day.

Cautions: Do not take drops undiluted. Discontinue or lower dosage if stomach irritation occurs.

GINKGO
Ginkgo biloba
Liquid extract of fresh, fall-harvested leaf.

Actions: Circulatory system tonic (esp. extremities, head and brain); optimizes brain cell metabolism; increases memory and learning capacity. PAF antagonist. Antioxidant. Valuable tonic for the aged.

Uses: Poor circulation in head and brain; memory loss, poor concentration and poor mental performance; Alzheimer's disease; dizziness and vertigo; degenerative eye disease; chronic inflammation in ears, and tinnitus ("ringing in ears"). Cold hands and feet; intermittent claudication and Raynaud's disease; varicose veins, leg ulcers and hemorrhoids. Male erectile dysfunction due to poor circulation. Asthma.

Dose: Take 30 to 40 drops, 3 to 5 times per day.

Cautions: Discontinue or lower dosage if headache occurs.

CHINESE GINSENG
Panax ginseng
Liquid extract of dried root.

Actions: Adaptogenic tonic that moderates harmful effects of stress (physical, mental/emotional, heat/cold and pollution); Enhances physical and mental energy, endurance, stamina and performance; improves sexual function, potency and fertility; Increases resistance to disease and speeds recuperation from illness. Withdrawal from drug addictions. Stomach tonic.

Uses: Excellent rejuvenating tonic (esp. for the aged). Debility and lack of physical and mental energy; chronic tiredness; nervous exhaustion; sexual debility. Weak immune system function. Moderates ill effects of radiation and chemotherapy. Chronic stomach problems.

Dose: Take 30 to 40 drops, 2 or 3 times per day.

Cautions: May cause sleeplessness if taken in evening. Do not take during acute infections or fevers.

SIBERIAN GINSENG
Eleutherococcus senticosus
Liquid extract of dried root.

Actions: Adaptogenic tonic that moderates harmful effects of stress (physical, mental/emotional, heat/cold and pollution); Enhances physical and mental energy, endurance, stamina and performance. Increases resistance to disease and speeds recuperation from illness.

Uses: Excellent rejuvenating tonic (esp. for the aged). Debility and lack of physical and mental energy; chronic tiredness; nervous exhaustion. Training aid for athletes. Weak immune system function. Moderates ill effects of radiation and chemotherapy. Withdrawal from drug addictions.

Dose: Take 30 to 40 drops, 2 to 3 times per day.

Cautions: May cause sleeplessness if taken in evening. Do not take during acute infections or fevers.

GOLDENROD
Solidago canadensis
Liquid extract of fresh flowering tops.

Actions: Soothing urinary system tonic; increases kidney function; diuretic. Mild anti-inflammatory and antispasmodic. Diaphoretic when taken in hot water.

Uses: Inflammation or infection of the genito-urinary tract; kidney pain; suppressed, difficult or scanty urination; back-ache associated with the kidneys; urinary stones or gravel; ulcerations of the bladder. Fevers.

Dose: Take 30 to 40 drops, 2 to 5 times per day.

Cautions: None known.

GOLDENSEAL
Hydrastis canadensis
Liquid extract of dried rhizome & rootlets.

Actions: Stimulating astringent; tonifies mucous membranes. Alterative. Stomach tonic and digestive bitters; improves appetite and digestion; promotes peristaltic action and muscular tone of stomach and intestines; promotes bile production. Antibacterial and antifungal. Uterine tonic.

Uses: Sub-acute and chronic inflammation of mucous membranes and glandular system with altered secretions; chronic inflammation and ulcerations of mouth and throat, nasal sinuses and pharynx, gastrointestinal system (e.g., gastric and duodenal ulcers, colitis), genito-urinary system (e.g., prolapsed uterus) and respiratory system (e.g., bronchial phlegm). Also indicated in passive bleeding from these tissues. Adjunct, long-range therapy for chronic constipation due to enfeebled relaxed tissues. Chronic atonic dyspepsia and poor digestion with torpid liver. Convalescence from protracted fevers and inflammation. Recovery from alcoholism and associated atonic gastrointestinal tract. Topically for infected wounds, ulcerations and bedsores, conjunctivitis ("pink eye"), etc.

Dose: Take 30 to 40 drops, 2 to 5 times per day. To enhance appetite and digestion take 15 minutes before meals. As a topical dressing or wash use full-strength (if well tolerated), or dilute with 2 or 3 parts water. For eye wash mix 3 to 10 drops in an eyecup filled with distilled water or saline solution and stir well with the glass dropper. Wash effected eye(s) for 1 minute, 1 to 3 times daily. If mixture stings uncomfortably, reduce number of extract drops to tolerance.

Cautions: Moderate use during pregnancy.

GOTU KOLA
Centella asiatica
Liquid extract of fresh whole herb with root..

Actions: Enhances integrity and vascularization of connective tissue and skin, hastens wound healing, and stimulates hair and nail growth. Improves elasticity and strength of blood vessels. Rejuvenating tonic.

Uses: Injury, disease and aging of the connective tissue and skin: Wounds, broken bones, torn ligaments and tendons, burns, anal fissures, ulcers (skin, stomach, duodenal, bladder and varicose), dermatitis, eczema, psoriasis, cellulitis, tendonitis, fibrocystic breast, liver cirrhosis, prevention and reduction of keloids and hypertrophic scars, leprosy, tuberculosis, lupus, scleroderma, periodontal (gum) disease, retinal detachment, tuberculosis, and varicose veins and hemorrhoids.

In the traditional Ayurvedic medicine of India, Gotu Kola is considered a Rasayana (rejuvenator) herb and has been used for centuries to increase vitality, prolong life and to enhance learning and memory.

Dose: Take 30 to 40 drops, 3 or 4 times per day. In severe conditions one can take up to 100 drops, 4 times per day.

Cautions: None known.

GRAVEL ROOT (Joe Pye Weed)
Eupatorium purpureum
Liquid extract of dried root

Actions: Mildly stimulating diuretic and astringent tonic that is very soothing to the urinary tract. Facilitates elimination of uric acid and prevents formation of urinary stones.

Uses: Chronic burning and irritation of urinary passages with constant urge to urinate (sense of obstruction), and painful, scanty, high-colored urine with mucous and blood. Excellent remedy in chronic cases of cystitis, urethritis, nephritis; urinary tract infections and catarrhs; tenesmus, strangury and stricture; albuminuria; prostatitis with boggy prostate, and benign prostate hypertrophy (BPH). Also useful in rheumatism, lumbago and gout. Excellent uterine tonic and "female remedy" indicated in chronic atony, irritability or displacement of uterus; chronic cases of endometritis, leukorrhea, amenorrhea and dysmenorrhea; and threatened miscarriage.

Dose: Take 30 to 40 drops, 3 to 4 times per day. Best given in hot water.

Cautions: None known.

GRINDELIA
Grindelia robusta
Liquid extract of dried flowers & leaf.

Actions: Respiratory stimulant and expectorant. Antiseptic, anti-inflammatory and vulnerary. Mild diuretic.

Uses: Harsh, dry, unproductive coughs with wheezing and constricted chest; asthmatic wheezing; bronchitis and sore bronchi. Removes detritus and mucous from kidney and urinary tract. Specific for swollen and congested spleen. Topically to treat wounds, indolent ulcers, impetigo, eczema, allergic dermatitis and poison ivy and poison oak.

Dose: Take 30 to 40 drops, 2 to 4 times per day. Topically apply full-strength (if well tolerated), or dilute with 2 or 3 parts water.

Cautions: May cause stomach irritation in larger doses.

HAWTHORN
Crataegus oxyacantha
Blended liquid extracts of dried spring-harvested
flowers & leaves, & autumn-harvested ripe berries.

Actions: Excellent nutritive, restorative tonic for heart and blood vessels; dilates coronary artery and improves blood flow to heart muscle; strengthens heart beat and regulates its rhythm; normalizes blood pressure. Excellent connective tissue tonic.

Uses: Specific for degenerative heart disease; arteriosclerosis; aging heart; smoker's heart; heart weakness due to debilitating or infectious disease; weak or irregular heart beat; high blood pressure. Degenerative or injured connective tissue (e.g., weak or injured ligaments and tendons, arthritic joints, varicose veins).

Dose: Take 30 to 40 drops, 2 to 3 times per day.

Cautions: Does not give quick results in emergencies; best results are seen with long-term use. Because Hawthorn may potentiate the effects of digitalis, patients on digitalis heart medication should consult with their physician before taking Hawthorn.

HOPS
Humulus lupulus
Liquid extract of dried, lupulin-rich strobiles.

Actions: Mild sedative. Bitter tonic that improves appetite and digestion. Contains significant amounts of phytoestrogens that have an estrogen-like action in the body.

Uses: Nervous agitation, restlessness, anxiety and hysteria; excellent in sleeplessness; alcoholic delirium tremens; nervous stomach and irritable bladder. Sexual over excitement and sexual neuroses (e.g., wet dreams, premature ejaculation); decreases abnormally high libido in men; priapism (persistent abnormal erection of penis).

Dose: Take 30 to 40 drops, 2 to 4 times per day. To enhance appetite and digestion take 15 minutes before meals.

Cautions: None known.

HOREHOUND

Marrubium vulgare

Liquid extract of dried leaf & flower.

Actions: Stimulant to all mucous membranes, but especially of the larynx and bronchi. Soothing expectorant and antispasmodic. Bitter digestive tonic and stomachic. Large doses can be laxative and emetic. Diaphoretic when taken hot.

Uses: Bronchitis; colds, flu and coughs (esp. non-productive coughs); chronic respiratory phlegm; asthma; hoarseness and laryngitis with loss of voice. Poor digestion due to atony of digestive system. Taken hot to bring on tardy menses.

Dose: Take 30 to 40 drops, 2 to 5 times per day. To enhance appetite and digestion take 15 minutes before meals.

Cautions: Moderate use during pregnancy.

HORSE CHESTNUT

Aesculus hippocastanum

Liquid extract of dry mature seed.

Actions: Reduces blood vessel permeability and thereby reduces vascular fragility and moderates inflammatory swelling; increases ability of blood vessels to reabsorb excess fluids from intercellular tissue spaces.

Uses: Reduces swelling caused by injury and inflammation: bruises, fractures, brain trauma and strokes; especially effective for varicose veins, spider veins, thrombophlebitis and hemorrhoids; chronic venous insufficiency (tiredness, heaviness, cramps, pain, itching and swelling in the legs); leg cramps at night; congested uterus and cervix; congestion of portal vessels.

Dose: Take 30 to 40 drops in half-cup of water, 2 to 4 times per day.

Cautions: None known.

HORSETAIL

Equisetum arvense

Liquid extract of fresh whole,
infertile herb, harvested in early spring.

Actions: Good source of soluble silica. Mild diuretic and urinary astringent. Slows or stops passive bleeding (internal and topical). Strengthens connective tissue.

Uses: Irritation, inflammation and passive bleeding of kidneys and urinary tract; urinary mucous discharge; urinary incontinence due to bladder irritation; suppressed urine; prostate gland inflammation. Edema. Passive bleeding of nose, stomach, intestines, lungs and bronchi. Repair of connective tissue: ulcers and slow-healing wounds; bone injury, osteoporosis and arthritic joint erosion; tuberculosis; chilblains.

Dose: Take 30 to 40 drops, 2 to 4 times per day. Topically apply full-strength (if well tolerated), or dilute with 2 or 3 parts water.

Cautions: None known.

HYDRANGEA
Hydrangea arborescens
Liquid extract of dried root.

Actions: Soothing, diuretic and tonic to membranes of genito-urinary systems; sedative to pain in kidneys, urethra and bladder; does not dissolve urinary stones but can prevent their formation and relieve irritation of formed stones. Soothing to membranes of respiratory passages.

Uses: Genito-urinary pain, irritation and congestion: acute inflammation of kidneys, bladder, urethra and prostate; frequent urination with quick, sharp, cutting pains and burning in bladder in urinary tract; difficult and painful urination; urinary tract pain after labor; tendency to form urinary stone; inflammation of prostate. Inflammation and irritation of respiratory passages.

Dose: Take 30 to 50 drops, 2 to 4 times per day. Best taken in hot water.

Cautions: None known.

JAMBUL (Java Plum)
Syzygium jambolanum
Liquid extract of mature seed.

Actions: This Aryuvedic herb has long been used to reduce the level of sugar in the blood and urine. Over a period of several weeks it can diminish the thirst associated with diabetes and decrease the quantity of urine output, and in some cases can lower the need for medical insulin. Also is a mild astringent, stomachic and pungent carminative.

Uses: Supportive therapy in the treatment of hyperglycemia and diabetes mellitus and associated symptoms of thirst and frequent urination. Diarrhea.

Dose: Take 30 to 40 drops, 2 to 5 times per day.

Cautions: Do not change the medical treatment of diabetes (esp. insulin dosage) without the advice of a qualified physician. Diabetics should monitor their blood sugar level and insulin dosage carefully while taking Jambul.

JUNIPER
Juniperus communis
Liquid extract of ovulate cone ("berry").

Actions: Aromatic resins serve as urinary stimulant, diuretic and antiseptic. Warming stimulant to digestive system; stomachic and carminative. Mild circulatory stimulant.

Uses: Chronic mucous discharge of genito-urinary system; gleet. Skin problems associated with torpid urinary system. Menstrual problems not associated with inflammation; emmenagogue for atonic amenorrhea. Chronic arthritis, gout and muscular rheumatic disease. Poor appetite and digestion due to atonic digestive system. Relief of flatulence. Topically for arthritic joints, sprains and strained muscles.

Dose: Take 30 to 40 drops, 2 or 3 times per day for no more than 6 weeks. Best used with soothing diuretics (e.g., Plantain, Marshmallow, Hydrangea). Topically apply full-strength over affected area.

Cautions: Moderate use during pregnancy. Avoid or moderate use in acute inflammation or pain of kidneys. Larger or prolonged doses (over six weeks) may irritate kidneys. Discontinue use if kidney irritation appears.

KAVA
Piper methysticum
Liquid extract of dried, 4 to 8 year-old rhizome & roots.

History: For 3,000 years South Pacific cultures have used Kava as a mild tranquilizer to relax the mind and clarify the thought processes, soothe the temperament, and induce a mild euphoria with feelings of peace and harmony. It is usually taken with a group to enhance sociability and evoke feelings of empathy and camaraderie, and is often used to settle disputes and facilitate reconciliation. In Europe Kava is an approved phytomedicine prescribed for anxiety and depression.

Actions: Excellent sedative, anti-anxiety, muscle relaxant, antispasmodic and anticonvulsive. Clarifies thought process and improves memory. Peaceful euphoriant. Analgesic and local anesthetic. Antiseptic (antifungal and antibacterial). Antiseptic diuretic.

Uses: Anxiety, despondency, nervousness and depression. Supportive therapy in anxiety-related diseases (e.g., asthma, high blood pressure), and with tremor (e.g., Parkinson's disease). Cramps and muscle spasms. Neuralgia (esp. trifacial nerve), toothache, earache and eye pain. Sleeplessness. Urinary infections; pain and spasms of urethra and bladder; painful urination. Premenstrual syndrome (PMS) and menstrual maladies. Lack of appetite. Topically as antifungal (e.g., ringworm, athletes foot).

Dose: Average dose is 30 to 40 drops taken 2 to 5 times per day. For more pronounced inducement of tranquility and euphoria, single doses up to 150 drops can be occasionally taken.

Cautions: Do not take Kava if taking psychiatric drugs, or when consuming alcohol. Kava is not a narcotic or intoxicant but excessive consumption may temporarily impair motor skills and ability to drive, or operate equipment. Large, frequent, long-continued doses can cause dry, itchy, scaly skin and bloodshot eyes. These symptoms soon disappear when Kava use is discontinued. Moderate use during pregnancy.

KHELLA
Ammi visnaga
Liquid extract of dried mature seed.

Actions: Smooth muscle relaxant and antispasmodic; non-stimulating bronchial dilator and vasodilator. Dilates urinary tract and sphincters, and the bile ducts. Dilates coronary artery, strengthens heart beat, and thereby enhances blood supply and metabolism of heart muscle.

Uses: Asthma, bronchitis and spastic coughs. Spasms and constriction of the urinary bladder and tract, and the gallbladder and bile duct; relieves urinary colic and facilitates discharge of urinary stones and thick mucous-pus discharge; relieves gallbladder colic and facilitates passage of gall stones. Indicated in coronary insufficiency, angina, arteriosclerosis, spastic heart, cardiac asthma, and recovery after heart attack. Does not increase heart rate or blood pressure. For spastic menstruation begin taking three to five days before expected period and continue until period ends.

Dose: Take 30 to 60 drops, 3 to 5 times per day.

In heart disease and asthma Khella may need to be taken for several weeks for positive effects. As effects persist for up to six hours, Khella is best used to prevent asthma attacks (esp. at night). Take 3 doses throughout the day and a dose before bed to assure a quiet night. Best combined with other respiratory antispasmodics (e.g., Skunk Cabbage, Lobelia, Thyme).

Cautions: Unreliable in acute asthma attacks or heart attacks. Avoid long exposure to sunlight or ultraviolet radiation while taking Khella.

LAVENDER
Lavandula vera
Liquid extract of dried flowers (no stems).

Actions: Pleasant aromatic and stomachic. Mild sedative and nerve tonic; anti-depressant.

Uses: Nervousness, anxiety, worry, depression. Sleeplessness; nightmares. Headache. Nervous stomach, nausea and motion sickness; indigestion.

Dose: Take 30 to 40 drops, 2 to 5 times per day.

Cautions: None known.

LEMON BALM
Melissa officinalis
Liquid extract of fresh leaf & flowering tops.

Actions: Pleasant aroma and taste; stomachic. Mild sedative and tranquilizer; antispasmodic. Promotes sweating (taken hot) and lowers fevers. Antiviral.

Uses: Nervous irritation; headaches; nervous heart; nervous stomach and indigestion with flatulence. Chills and fevers. Menstrual blues and emotions. Herpes (used internally and topically) and other viral diseases. Excellent remedy for babies and young children: colds, flu and fevers; teething; nervousness, over-excitment, peevishness and sleeplessness; colic.

Dose: Take 30 to 40 drops, 2 to 5 times per day. Take in hot water for fevers. Topically apply full-strength.

Cautions: None known.

LICORICE
Glycyrrhiza glabra var. *typica*
Liquid extract of dried, unpeeled root & stolon.

Actions: Demulcent and soothing to mucous membranes; expectorant. Antiviral. Anti-inflammatory. Liver protective. Adrenal gland tonic. Mildly laxative in large doses. Sweet-tasting corrigent.

Uses: Soothing coughs and clearing phlegm; bronchitis, laryngitis and pharyngitis. Stomach inflammation and ulcers; colitis. Adrenal gland insufficiency. Liver inflammation and hepatitis.

Dose: Take 30 to 40 drops, 2 to 5 times per day. Larger doses can be taken, but for no longer that 4 weeks.

Cautions: Excessive, long-continued doses can cause potassium loss and water retention, headaches and high blood pressure. These symptoms cease when Licorice is discontinued. Excessive or long-continued doses are contraindicated in high blood pressure and congestive heart disease.

LINDEN
Tilia cordata & *T. platyphyllos*
Liquid extract of dried flower with bract.

Actions: Sedative and antispasmodic; hypotensive. Diuretic. Diaphoretic. Mild astringent.

Uses: Fevers, colds and flu; coughs. Nervous tension and headaches. High blood pressure. Diarrhea. Excellent remedy for children.

Dose: Take 30 to 40 drops, 2 to 4 times per day. To induce sweat during fevers, take drops in hot water.

Cautions: None known.

MARSHMALLOW
Althaea officinalis
Liquid extract of fresh root.

Actions: Very mucilagenous and demulcent; expectorant; mild astringent. Soothing to gastrointestinal, bronchi and urinary tracts. Enhances immune system response.

Uses: Inflammation and irritation of membranes of gastrointestinal, bronchi and urinary tracts; dry coughs; dry sore throat; stomach ulcers; diarrhea; cystitis and burning urine. Weak immune system.

Dose: Take 30 to 60 drops, 2 to 5 times per day.

Cautions: None known.

MEADOWSWEET
Spirea ulmaria
Liquid extract of dried leaf & flowering tops (no stem).

Actions: Meadowsweet's high content of aspirin-like compounds (salicylic aldehyde and methyl salicylate) makes it an excellent analgesic and antirheumatic without the side-effects of aspirin. It is aromatic, anti-inflammatory, astringent, diuretic (taken with cool water) and diaphoretic (taken with hot water); is also stomachic and a gastric antacid which soothes stomach mucosa and normalizes its secretions.

Uses: Minor pains; arthritis, and rheumatic joint and muscle pains; headache; toothache; sprains and tendinitis; and topically for insect stings. Fevers, colds and flu. Acid dyspepsia ("heartburn"), gastritis; eructation and esophageal burning; stomach ulcers. Aromatic astringent for diarrhea (esp. with children). Mild urinary antiseptic indicated in irritation, inflammation and infections of the urinary passage; acute catarrhal cystitis; gleet; prostatic enlargement and prostatorrhea; chronic cervicitis and vaginitis with leukorrheal discharge.

Dose: Take 30 to 40 drops, 2 to 5 times per day. For diarrhea take up to 1 teaspoon of extract mixed into a cup of water (for children's dose, see Clark's Rule, pg. 128).

Cautions: None known.

MILK THISTLE
Silybum marianum
Liquid extract of dried mature seed.

Actions: Hepatoprotective (protects liver from toxins) and liver restorative. Tonic to spleen. Rich in antioxidant flavonoids. Vascular tonic.

Uses: Inflammatory, infectious and degenerative liver diseases. Protects liver from toxic drugs, chemicals and pollutants. Swollen spleen. Supportive therapy for asthma. Degenerative disorders of blood vessels; varicose veins; hemorrhoids.

Dose: Take 30 to 40 drops, 2 to 4 times per day.

Cautions: None known.

MUIRA PUAMA (Potency Wood)
Ptychopetalum olacoides
Liquid extract of dried stem with bark.

Actions: Soothing nervous system tonic. Enhances sexual libido in men and women. Aromatic stomachic and carminative. Antirheumatic.

Uses: Sexual weakness, impotency or performance anxiety in men, and lack of sexual desire or frigidity in women. Premenstrual syndrome (PMS), and menstrual cramps. Neurasthenia (nervous exhaustion) and nervous depression. Neuralgia. Adjunct therapy in arthritis and rheumatism. Nervous stomach and diarrhea.

Dose: As a tonic take 30 to 60 drops, 2 or 3 times per day. As stimulant take 60 drops in hot water.

Cautions: None known.

MULLEIN
Verbascum thapsus & *V. olympicum*
Blended liquid extracts of fresh leaf, flower & bud.

Actions: Soothing expectorant. Soothing demulcent to lymphatics and mucous membranes. Soothing diuretic.

Uses: Inflammation of respiratory and urinary passages; dry coughs and hoarseness; cystitis and burning urine. Sores in mouth and throat. Diarrhea. Lymphatic irritation and swellings; mumps. Moderates stronger-acting lymphatic herbs (e.g., Poke root).

Dose: Take 30 to 60 drops, 2 to 5 times per day.

Cautions: None known.

MYRRH
Commiphora abyssinica
Liquid extract of oleo-gum-resin masses ("tears").

Actions: Astringent, antiseptic, anti-inflammatory and vulnerary. Stimulant to blood circulation. Warming digestive bitters and stomachic. Stimulating, antiseptic expectorant. Classic remedy for mouth and gums. Specific for conditions that produce pus.

Uses: Torpid mucous membranes with ulcerations and excessive tenacious mucous; as spray or swab for spongy membranes and ulcerations of mouth, gums, tonsils, pharynx and nasal cavity; sore throat. Chronic inflammation, congestion and mucous discharge of urinary tract, bronchi, uterus and vagina; gleet. Poor appetite and digestion (taken before meals). Poor circulation with cold skin. Topically applied to cold sores and herpes, indolent ulcers and infected wounds. Respiratory infections and bronchitis with excess mucous.

Dose: Take 20 to 40 drops in a little water, 2 to 4 times per day. To enhance appetite and digestion take 15 minutes before meals. Topically apply full-strength (if well tolerated), or dilute with 2 or 3 parts water or glycerine. As gargle, mix drops in a little water and gargle several times per day.

Cautions: Large doses may irritate stomach.

NETTLE
Urtica dioica
Blended extracts of fresh flowering
tops, fresh root and dry mature seed.

Actions: Nutritive, alterative tonic. Antihistamine and anti-inflammatory; moderates allergic response. Urinary tonic and diuretic. Astringent to mucous membranes. Hemostatic. Galactagogue.

Uses: Chronic inflammations, excessive mucous discharge and ulcerations of the mucous membranes; burning or difficult urination; allergies with stinging, runny nose and eyes; hemorrhoids; swollen prostate and benign prostatic hypertrophy (BPH). Inflammations, eruptions and rashes of skin; hives, eczema, psoriasis, chicken pox (esp. if hot and stinging). Arthritis and gout. Passive bleeding in all parts of body; profuse menstruation. Suppressed milk flow in nursing mothers. Topically applied to eczema, poison ivy, rashes and insect stings.

Dose: Take 30 to 40 drops, 2 to 5 times per day. For topical use mix half-and-half with rosewater and apply freely to troubled area.

Cautions: None known.

OAT SEED
Avena sativa
Liquid extract of fresh,
immature seed harvested in the "milky" stage.

Actions: Restorative nerve and heart tonic.

Uses: Neurasthenia (nervous depletion) and nervous breakdown; worry, anxiety and depression; nervous insomnia. Sexual depletion or exhaustion. Enfeebled heart. To aid convalescence after debilitating disease. Support withdrawal from tobacco and other drug addictions; delirium tremens.

Dose: Take 30 to 40 drops, 2 to 5 times per day.

Cautions: Avoid use of Oat Seed Extract if you are allergic to Oats.

OLIVE LEAF
Olea europaea
Liquid extract of dried leaf.

Actions: Broad-spectrum antiviral. Dilates coronary artery and regulates heartbeat. Lowers blood pressure. Lowers cholesterol in blood.

Uses: Virus infections, including flu and herpes. General heart tonic; irregular heart beat (arrhythmia). High blood pressure. Hypercholesterol.

Dose: Take 30 to 40 drops, 2 to 4 times per day.

Cautions: None known.

PEPPERMINT SPIRITS
Mentha piperita
Liquid extract of dried leaf blended with essential oil of fresh herb.

Actions: Stomachic that enhances circulation and secretions of stomach; stomach antispasmodic and carminative; relieves nausea and vomiting; checks abnormal fermentation in stomach. Breath freshener. Flavorful, aromatic corrigent.

Uses: Agreeable taste makes Peppermint especially useful in various maladies of the stomach, and, to a lesser degree, the intestines: stomach upset, gastro-intestinal spasms, flatulent colic; to allay nausea and vomiting and ease diarrhea discomfort. Promotes good digestion and relieves indigestion. Eases griping caused by laxatives. Excellent adjunct in treating gastro-intestinal symptoms associated with maladies of the gall bladder and pancreas. Excellent, quick-acting remedy for hiccup. Produces sweating and promotes recovery from colds and flu (taken in hot water). Taken internally and rubbed into the temples and forehead, it gives relief from nervous headaches, migraines and sick headaches.

Dose: Take 20 to 40 drops in half-cup water, 2 to 5 times per day. Best taken after meals to facilitate good digestion or relieve indigestion.

Cautions: When applying topically, take care not to get the extract or its vapors in the eyes.

PETASITES
Petasites officinalis

Liquid extract of fresh rhizome (pyrrolizidine alkaloids removed).

Actions: Antispasmodic. Soothing, demulcent, expectorant and antitussive. Sedative and analgesic.

Uses: General coughs, whooping cough, bronchitis, laryngitis, pharyngitis. Asthma. Especially indicated in chronic spasmodic coughs. Muscle spasms; acute spasms and pain of urinary tract and gallbladder; nervous stomach; menstrual cramps. Headaches and migraines. Low back pain. Eases pain in certain cancers.

Dose: Take 30 to 40 drops, 2 to 5 times per day. As expectorant, is best taken in hot water or tea.

Cautions: Avoid Petasites preparations containing pyrrolizidine alkaloids.

PRICKLY ASH
Xanthoxylum clava-herculis

Liquid extract of dried tree bark.

Actions: Stimulating alterative tonic to circulatory system and nervous systems (does not excite or agitate), and enhances secretions and general metabolism. Stimulates flow of saliva and digestive juices, increases appetite and enhances digestion; carminative. Enhances immune system function; antirheumatic. Diaphoretic.

Uses: All conditions of marked atony and deficient secretions; torpor and catarrh of mucous membranes; chronic dyspepsia and catarrhal gastritis; flatulent colic. Sluggish blood and lymphatic circulation; cold skin and extremities; intermittent claudication and Raynaud's syndrome. Alterative in skin diseases (e.g., eczema, psoriasis). Weak nerve force. Sexual problems associated wih chronic torpor of sexual glands and organs. To potentiate action of other immune system herbs (e.g., Echinacea, Burdock). Arthritis, rheumatism and gout. Tonic in slow recuperation from depleting illness. Fevers, colds and flu.

Dose: Take 30 to 40 drops, 2 to 4 times per day.

Cautions: None known.

RED ROOT

Ceanothus americanus

Liquid extract of dry whole root.

Actions: Tonic, astringent and stimulant to mucous membranes; expectorant. Glandular alterative which promotes decongestion in the portal circulation, lymphatic tissue, liver, and especially the spleen. Facilitates drainage of cysts and swollen glands.

Uses: Swollen lymph nodes and adenoids; sore throat, pharyngitis and tonsillitis; mumps; mononucleosis; chronic torpor of stomach and liver; swollen, congested liver. Excellent remedy for enlarged, congested spleen (esp. of malarial origin) and chronic or sub-acute splenitis. Clears catarrhal conditions with excessive, thick secretions; chronic bronchitis. Ovarian cysts.

Dose: Take 30 to 40 drops, 2 to 4 times per day.

Cautions: Not to be used in acute splenitis; use only after acute symptoms have passed and pressure to spleen does not markedly aggravate the pain.

SAW PALMETTO

Serenoa repens

Liquid extract of semi-dried berry.

Actions: Restorative sexual tonic for men and women. Antiandrogenic effect on prostate gland. Relaxes and soothes the urinary tract, and improves urinary outflow. Anti-inflammatory and immunomodulator.

Uses: Excellent remedy in benign prostatic hypertrophy (BPH) and related urinary maladies (urine slow to start, incomplete urination, frequent nighttime urination). Inflammation of genito-urinary organs and vessels; urethritis; prostatitis; enlarged uterus. Retarded physical and sexual maturation in adolescents; underdeveloped prostate, testes, breasts, ovaries or uterus; inability to gain weight. Male baldness. Physical masculinization of women (excessive body hair, underdeveloped breasts).

Dose: Take 30 to 40 drops, 2 to 5 times per day.

Cautions: Rarely causes nausea.

SKULLCAP
Scutellaria lateriflora
Liquid extract of fresh flowering herb.

Actions: Restorative nerve tonic and mild sedative. Antispasmodic

Uses: Nervous exhaustion and neurasthenia; mental overwork; nervous breakdown and depression; nerve depletion due to depleting disease. Irritation of nervous system; nervous agitation, hysteria and anxiety; rage and anger; nervous tremor. Nervous heart disorders. Support therapy in epilepsy. Insomnia. Withdrawal from alcohol and other drug addictions; delirium tremens.

Dose: Take 30 to 40 drops, 2 to 4 times per day.

Cautions: Beware of adulteration of Skullcap with Germander herb (Teucrium chamaedrys).

SPILANTHES
Spilanthes achmella & *S. oleracea*
Liquid extract of fresh whole flowering herb with root.

Actions: Stimulating alterative tonic. Enhances immune system function; antibacterial, antifungal, antiviral; antimalarial. Because of their high isobutylamide content, Spilanthes and Prickly Ash have similar stimulating and therapeutic actions (see Prickly Ash).

Uses: General infection fighter. Fungus infections: candida, thrush, ringworm, athlete's foot. Cold sores and herpes. Colds, flu and respiratory infections; ear infections. Prevention and treatment of malaria and Lyme's disease. Diminished secretions of mucous membranes.

Dose: Take 30 to 40 drops, 2 to 5 times per day. Topically apply fullstrength (if well tolerated), or dilute with 1 or 2 parts water.

Cautions: None known.

ST. JOHN'S WORT
Hypericum perforatum
Liquid extract of fresh flowering & budding tops.

Actions: Increases life and potentiates effects of neurotransmitters. Nerve tonic; mild sedative and antidepressant. Antiviral against HIV and hepatitis C. Vulnerary (esp. to inflamed or injured nerves).

Uses: Nervous debility, anxiety and mental depression; anorexia. Nerve injury, inflammation and pain: brain concussion, shock or injury of spine or soreness of spinal area; sciatica; multiple sclerosis; shingles (taken internally and topically). Topically to treat trauma soreness, wounds, bruises, contusions and shingles.

Dose: Take 30 to 40 drops, 2 to 5 times per day. Topically apply full-strength (if well tolerated), or dilute with 1 or 2 parts water.

Cautions: Avoid intense or prolonged exposure to sunlight or ultraviolet light while taking St. John's Wort extract.

STONE ROOT
Collinsonia canadensis
Liquid extract of fresh flowering tops & rhizome.

Actions: Heart and circulatory tonic; quiets irritation and gives strength and regularity to heart's action. Astringent tonic to veins and mucous membranes; allays venous stasis, congestion and sense of constriction in the throat, larynx and ears.

Uses: Specific to maladies associated with flaccid, atonic veins, venous stasis and torpor of portal circulation: hemorrhoids with constriction, heat and weight in rectum (esp. during pregnancy); to relieve soreness and facilitate recovery from rectal surgery; varicose veins; vascular engorgement and mucous membrane irritation of pelvic viscera (e.g., chronic gastro-enteritis with catarrh or diarrhea). Female disorders dependent upon varicosis: amenorrhea, dysmenorrhea, menorrhagia, leukorrhea, flaccid or prolapsed uterus and threatened miscarriage. Chronic laryngitis, pharyngitis, middle-ear inflammation, bronchitis and tracheitis; hoarseness due to voice strain. Heart debility due to inflammation, protracted fevers and overstrain, and in chronic inflammation of pericardium. Chronic catarrhal conditions of kidneys and bladder.

Dose: Take 30 to 40 drops, 2 to 4 times per day. As gargle mix drops in a little water and gargle several times per day.

Cautions: None known.

USNEA
Usnea barbata

Liquid extract of dried tree lichen extracted with hot alcohol.

Actions: Usnea's usnic acid has shown effective anti-microbial activity against fungus, trichomonas protozoa, gram-positive bacteria (e.g., Staphylococcus, Streptococcus, and Pneumonococcus, including penicillin resistant strains), and tuberculosis bacillus. Usnic acid shows no antimicrobial activity against gram-negative bacteria (e.g., E. coli and Salmonella). Increases resistance against colds and flu.

Uses: Fungus infections (e.g., candidiasis, athlete's foot, ringworm); boils; impetigo; mastitis; bronchial infections and pneumonia; sore throat or strep throat (gargle); sinus infections (diluted spray); skin and lung tuberculosis; trichomoniasis; dysentery (but not typhoid, cholera or other intestinal infections caused by gram-negative bacteria). Especially effective against urinary tract infections and upper respiratory infections.

Dose: Take 30 to 40 drops, 2 to 5 times per day. Topically apply full-strength (if well tolerated), or dilute with 1 or 2 parts water. As gargle mix drops in a little water and gargle several times per day. As nasal spray mix 15 to 25 drops in half-cup saline solution and use 2 to 4 times per day.

Cautions: None known.

VIOLET (Heartsease)
Viola tricolor

Liquid extract of fresh flowering plant.

Actions: Soothing, demulcent expectorant and diuretic. Lowers fevers. Mild sedative. Gentle and effective alterative for babies and young children.

Uses: General infections, fever, colds, flu and coughs. Skin eruptions, hives, eczema, cradle-cap and milk-crust. Smelly, staining or burning urine. Violet is especially indicated, and is very safe for babies and young children.

Dose: Adults can take 30 to 40 drops, 2 to 5 times per day. Lower dosage according to body weight for children (see Clark's Rule, pg. 128).

Cautions: None known.

WILD INDIGO
Baptisia tinctoria
Liquid extract of fresh, non-woody root.

Actions: Stimulating, antiseptic alterative which especially influences the glandular and lymphatic systems. Enhances anabolic and catabolic metabolism. Stimulant to liver and bowels. A specific remedy in atonic conditions associated with weak vitality, feeble capillary circulation, fetid excretions, and sepsis with tendency towards breakdown, ulceration, and necrosis of tissue. Especially indicated in conditions showing fullness of tissue with dusky leaden hue, fetor and tendency to sloughing or ulceration.

Uses: Toxemia and septicemia ("blood poisoning") with associated fetid breath; fetid discharges of wounds, ulcerations or tumors, and of ears, nose, vagina, bowels, etc.; eruptive fevers, and asthenic fevers with depressed vitality (esp. typhoid); adverse reactions to inoculations; enlarged, congested lymph nodes; mononucleosis; boils; mouth sores and spongy gums; septic sore throat, tonsillitis, pharyngitis and quinsy; inflammation of nasal membranes with ulceration and discharge; intestinal toxemia or dysentery with putrid stools; gastric or duodenal ulcers, ulcerative colitis and ulcerations of Peyer's patches; fetid leucorrhea, and ulcerated or eroded cervix or os; inflamed breasts; indolent surface ulcers with bluish edges; gangrene.

Dose: Take 30 to 40 drops, 3 to 4 times per day for no longer than 6 weeks. Topically apply full-strength (if well tolerated), or dilute with 1 or 2 parts water. As gargle mix drops in a little water and gargle several times per day. Wild Indigo is best taken with Echinaea and Myrrh.

Cautions: Moderate use during pregnancy. Lower dosage or discontinue use if nausea or diarrhea occur.

WILD YAM
Dioscorea villosa
Liquid extract of dry whole rhizome.

Actions: Antispasmodic, especially to genito-urinary and gastro-intestinal systems. Diaphoretic (taken in hot water).

Uses: Relief of nervous system irritation. Abdominal cramps, pain and tenderness; spastic colics (esp. gallbladder colic); flatulent colic; spastic colitis; spasmodic pain in uterus, cervix or ovaries; menstrual cramps; after-pains of labor. Nausea and vomiting during pregnancy. Early stages of peritonitis.

Dose: Take 30 to 40 drops, 2 to 5 times per day. In spastic conditions give 20 drops in warm water every half-hour. If relief is not seen within 2 hours the remedy is probably not going to work.

Cautions: May cause nausea with larger doses.

YARROW
Achillea millefolium
Liquid extract of dry flowers.

Actions: Astringent and hemostatic; vascular tonic. Diaphoretic and anti-fever. Antiseptic vulnerary. Aromatic digestive bitters.

Uses: Excellent for inducing sweat and lowering fevers (taken in hot water); colds and flu. Passive bleeding and excessive menstrual flow. Astringent to atonic relaxed tissues with free discharges and tendency to ulceration; diarrhea; atonic uterus and leucorrhoea. Varicose veins and hemorrhoids. Stimulates appetite and improves digestion.

Dose: Take 30 to 40 drops, 2 to 5 times per day. To enhance appetite and digestion take 15 minutes before meals.

Cautions: May cause nausea with larger doses.

YOHIMBE
Corynanthe yohimbe
Liquid extract of dried tree bark.

Actions: Sexual stimulant to men and women that increases libido (aphrodisiac). Stimulates erectile tissue in both sexes, and enhances sexual sensitivity, arousal and orgasm. Increases sperm production and motility.

Uses: Low sex drive or response in both sexes. Male erectile dysfunction; low sperm count.

Dose: As general, non-stimulating tonic take 30 to 40 drops, 2 or 3 times per day for no longer than 6 weeks. Best taken with sexual tonics (e.g., Ginseng, Oat Seed). As sexual stimulant, larger more frequent doses may be taken, but only with caution (see below).

Cautions: Can cause nervousness, sleeplessness, anxiety, tremor, increased blood pressure and tachycardia; discontinue use if these symptoms appear. Avoid excessive or long-term use. Do not give to children, the aged or pregnant women. Contraindicated in inflammation of sexual organs and glands; heart, blood pressure and kidney disease; in gastric and duodenal ulcers; in diabetes; with psychiatric patients or with mood-modifying drugs such as antidepressants

HERBAL
COMPOUNDS

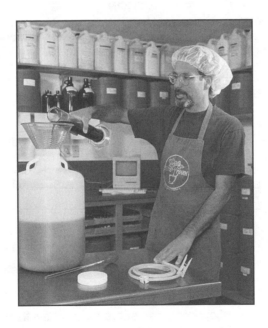

ANGELICA • DEVIL'S CLAW COMPOUND
Arthritis & Gout Remedy

A blend of the liquid extracts of:
- **Devil's Claw tuber** (Harpagophytum procumbens)   22.5%
- **Jamaican Sarsaparilla root** (Smilax ornata)   22.5%
- **Nettle mature seed** (Urtica dioica)   20.0%
- **Burdock mature seed** (Arctium lappa)   20.0%
- **Angelica root** (Angelica archangelica)   7.5%
- **Prickly Ash bark** (Xanthoxylum clava-herculis)   7.5%
  - Dried

ACTION
The anti-inflammatory, antioxidant, and immunopotentiating actions of this compound make it a specific in the treatment of inflammatory joint diseases by preventing or minimizing inflammatory damage to synovial membranes, cartilage and other joint tissues. Also, this compound can help remove uric acid crystals from joints and other tissues by lowering the concentration of uric acid in the blood and facilitating its excretion by the kidneys.

USES
A specific in the treatment of **rheumatoid arthritis** and **gout**. Although this compound can be helpful in **osteoarthritis** (more accurately called osteoarthrosis or degenerative joint disease), it is not as specifically indicated here because osteoarthritis is primarily a degenerative disorder with little or no inflammation.

DOSE
Acute: Three to five times per day take 30 to 50 drops in a little water.

Chronic: Three times per day take 20 to 40 drops in a little water.

ADJUNCT THERAPY
TURMERIC•CHAMOMILE COMPOUND can serve as an anti-inflammatory booster in acute or persistent cases of rheumatoid arthritis and gout. Add 30 to 50 drops to each dose of the above.

Use ECHINACEA EXTRACT to enhance immune response in rheumatoid arthritis, osteoarthritis, and *chronic* gout. *Do not* take Echinacea during acute attacks of gout. Three to five times per day take 30 to 40 drops in water. Can be mixed and taken with the above doses.

Use BLACK COHOSH EXTRACT to relieve the constricted muscles around inflamed joints. Three to four times per day take 30 to 40 drops in water. Can be mixed and taken with the above doses.

THUJA•GOTU KOLA COMPOUND may be helpful as a restorative to the connective tissue of the joints (depending upon the degree of deterioration). Three times per day take 30 to 40 drops in water. Best taken one to two hours before or after the above doses.

HERBAL LINIMENT can be applied topically over the affected joint(s) to relieve pain and to improve local circulation. Apply as described under *Herbal Liniment*.

COLCHICUM AUTUMNALE EXTRACT is one of the oldest and most effective herbal remedies for gout but, because of its potential toxicity, it must be administered by a qualified physician.

CAUTIONS

Certain types of arthritis (e.g., progenic & tuberculous arthritis) can be very damaging in a short period of time. Therefore early diagnosis and treatment is imperative to prevent permanent damage.

Arthritis should be properly diagnosed and treated by a qualified healthcare practitioner.

AVENA • LICORICE COMPOUND

Tobacco Addiction Remedy

A blend of the liquid extracts of:

★ **Oat "milky" seed** (Avena sativa)   30%
● **Licorice root** (Glycyrrhiza glabra)   25%
● **Lobelia herb, & seed** (Lobelia inflata)   20%
● **Sassafras root bark** (Sassafras officinale)   15%
● **Calamus rhizome** (Acorus calamus)   10%

★ Fresh   ● Dried

ACTION

Recent research has shown that tincture of fresh (undried) Oat can facilitate withdrawal from tobacco and opium addiction.

The alkaloid *lobeline,* which is found in Lobelia, has a chemical structure and physiological effects that are similar to *nicotine,* and is believed to mask the withdrawal symptoms of nicotine addiction without itself being addictive.

USES

Indicated in the treatment of **tobacco *(nicotine)* addiction.** Lessens the desire for nicotine, supports the nervous system and the adrenal glands, and has a cleansing and restorative action on the lungs and bronchi.

DOSE

Three to five times per day take 20 to 30 drops in water.

ADJUNCT THERAPY

In case of nervous withdrawal symptoms take 20 to 40 drops of AVENA • SKULLCAP COMPOUND with each dose of the above.

CAUTIONS

Because of the Lobelia in this compound, large and frequent doses may induce nausea or vomiting in some sensitive individuals. If this happens, discontinue use for 1 or 2 days, and then resume use with a lower number of drops. Drops can be adjusted according to tolerance.

AVENA • SKULLCAP COMPOUND
Restorative Nerve Tonic

A blend of the liquid extracts of:
* ★ **Skullcap flowering herb** (Scutellaria lateriflora)   25%
* ★ **Oat "milky" seed** (Avena sativa)   25%
* ★ **St. John's Wort flower & bud** (Hypericum perf.)   20%
* • **Celery whole plant, & seed** (Apium graveolens)   15%
* • **Lavender flower** (Lavandula vera)   15%

★ Fresh   • Dried

ACTION
While this compound has a mild sedative action, it primarily serves as a restorative tonic to the entire nervous system.

USES
Indicated in nervous affections associated with low or exhausted nerve force. It is a specific for **neurasthenia** ("nervous exhaustion") and nerve weakness which is the result of severe or prolonged illness or stress ("I just can't seem to get my energy back"). It can be helpful in **"nervous breakdown,"** **depression**, **"jittery nerves,"** **nervous heart** disorders, restlessness and mental fatigue, **delirium tremens** and **drug withdrawal** (marijuana, alcohol, tobacco, coffee, cocaine, heroin, etc.). This compound may also be helpful as adjunct therapy in the treatment of epilepsy, multiple sclerosis & Parkinson's disease.

DOSE
Three to five times per day take 20 to 40 drops in water. Take last drops of the day just before bed. For optimal results take for 1 to 3 months.

ADJUNCT THERAPY
As a general tonic to relieve the physical & mental fatigue associated with stress and worry, take 25 to 40 drops of SIBERIAN GINSENG EXTRACT 2 or 3 times per day. If sleeplessness results, do not take at night.

CAUTIONS
As this compound contains alcohol, it would not be indicated in the treatment of alcoholics who have ceased the intake of all alcohol.

Some of the maladies listed above can be serious health problems and will require treatment by a qualified healthcare practitioner.

BLACK COHOSH • LICORICE COMPOUND
Estrogen Enhancing Tonic

A blend of the liquid extracts of:
- **Black Cohosh rhizome & roots** (Cimicifuga racemosa) 20%
- **Chaste Tree berry** (Vitex agnus-castus) 20%
- **Saw Palmetto berry** (Serenoa serrulata) 20%
- **Sage leaf** (Salvia officinalis) 20%
- **Licorice root** (Glycyrrhiza glabra) 20%
  - Dried

ACTION
Black Cohosh, Saw Palmetto, Sage & Licorice contain phytoestrogens (estrogen-like compounds) which, when taken into the body, mimic the chemistry of estrogen. Their estrogen activity is much slower & weaker than that of medical estrogen, but is free of estrogen's side effects.

USES
As supportive therapy in cases of **female hypogonadism** and **chronic estrogen deficiency**. Its use may be helpful in maladies related to estrogen deficiency: menopause, failure of pituitary gland to stimulate development of secondary sex characteristics, postpartum breast engorgement, and to initiate menstrual periods and relieve secondary amenorrhea.

DOSE
Three times per day take 30 to 40 drops in a little water, in cycles of three weeks on and one week off.

ADJUNCT THERAPY
Concentrated alfalfa juice powder (but not alfalfa sprouts) and soy foods (e.g., tofu, temphe, soy milk) are excellent sources of phytoestrogens.

Pomegranates contain small amounts of natural estrogen. Eat the ripe fruit or juice as desired.

CAUTIONS
In some women the estrogen activity of this compound may not be strong enough to successfully treat their estrogen deficiency. Anyone who is taking medically prescribed estrogen should not substitute with this compound without first consulting with their physician.

BUGLEWEED • MOTHERWORT COMPOUND
Hyperthyroid Remedy

A blend of the liquid extracts of:
- **Bugleweed flowering herb** (Lycopus virginicus) 30%
- **Motherwort flowering tops** (Leonurus cardiaca) 30%
- ★ **Cactus flower & stem** (Selenicereus grandiflorus) 20%
- ★ **Lemon Balm leaf & flower** (Melissa officinalis) 20%

★ Fresh   • Dried

ACTION
Thyroxine antagonist. Moderates an overactive thyroid gland. General sedative which soothes a nervous or excitable heart.

USES
Hyperthyroidism (overactive thyroid gland). Especially indicated when hyperthyroid condition is associated with nervous, overactive heart with palpitations or tachycardia.

DOSE
Three to five times per day take 30 to 50 drops in water.

ADJUNCT THERAPY
To further support the heart, take 30 to 40 drops of HAWTHORN EXTRACT with each dose of the above.

For associated nervousness or tremor take 30 to 40 drops of AVENA • SKULLCAP COMPOUND with each dose of the above

For associated sleeplessness take VALERIAN • PASSIONFLOWER COMPOUND as directed.

CAUTIONS
Hyperthyroidism can be a serious, life-threatening disease and should be treated under the care of a qualified health care practitioner.

This herbal compound may not be compatible with drugs used to treat hyperthyroidism. Consult your healthcare practitioner before mixing the two.

BURDOCK • SARSAPARILLA COMPOUND

Skin Remedy for Eczema, Psoriasis, Acne, etc.

A blend of the liquid extracts of:

• **Burdock mature seed** (Arctium lappa)	18%
• **Jamaican Sarsaparilla root** (Smilax ornata)	18%
• **Nettle mature seed** (Urtica dioica)	18%
• **Yellow Dock root** (Rumex crispus)	18%
★ **Spilanthes flowering herb** (Spilanthes oleracea)	18%
• **Sassafras root bark** (Sassafras officinale)	10%

★ Fresh • Dried

ACTION

The alterative, depurative, anti-inflammatory, and immunopotentiating actions of this compound make it a specific in the treatment of many skin diseases, especially those associated with autotoxemia.

USES

This compound is specific in the treatment of **atopic dermatitis (eczema)**, **psoriasis**, **acne**, and **seborrhea & dandruff**. It can also be very helpful as adjunct therapy in the treatment of **contact dermatitis**, **stasis dermatitis**, **actinic dermatitis** ("sun poisoning"), **neurodermatitis** ("nervous eczema"), and **ichthyosis**.

DOSE

Acute: Three to five times per day take 30 to 50 drops in water.

Chronic: Three times per day take 30 to 40 drops in water.

ADJUNCT THERAPY

TURMERIC • CHAMOMILE COMPOUND serves as an anti-inflammatory booster in acute or persistent inflammatory dermatitis. Add 30 to 50 drops to each dose of the above.

BLUE FLAG EXTRACT is indicated in dermatitides associated with oily or "greasy" skin (e.g., acne or seborrhea). **Adults:** Three times per day take 5 to 15 drops in at least 8 ounces of water. **Children:** Only give Blue Flag to children 12 years old or older, and then only as calculated by Clark's Rule. Lower dosage or discontinue use if drops cause nausea, diarrhea or G.I. tract irritation.

VIOLA TRICOLOR EXTRACT is specific for "cradle cap" and eczema of infants. Three times per day give in water, juice or milk, 1 drop per 4 pounds of child's body weight (e.g. 5 drops for a 20-pound child).

COLLINSONIA • HORSE CHESTNUT COMPOUND is recommended in the treatment of **stasis dermatitis** to facilitate venous return and relieve tissue edema. Three times per day take 30 to 40 drops in water.

CAUTIONS

Many skin maladies are symptoms of other disorders inside the body. Therefore, to properly treat skin disease, it is necessary to determine and treat any underlying disorders.

Although dermatitis is seldom dangerous, certain forms (e.g., exfoliative dermatitis) can be life-threatening. Therefore, it is important that dermatitis be properly diagnosed and treated by a qualified healthcare practitioner.

CACTUS • HAWTHORN COMPOUND
Cardiovascular Tonic

A blend of the liquid extracts of:
- **Hawthorn berry, leaf & flower** (Crataegus oxy.)   35%
- ★ **Cactus flower & stem** (Selenicereus grandiflorus) 30%
- **Motherwort leaf & flower** (Leonurus cardiaca)   25%
- **Ginger rhizome** (Zingiber officinale)   10%

★ Fresh   • Dried

ACTION
Hawthorn's flavonoids have been shown to enhance the connective tissue structure of the endothelial lining of the heart cavities and the blood & lymph vessels, thus optimizing their resiliency against the damages of injury, disease, stress, and aging. Hawthorn dilates the coronary artery and thereby enhances blood flow to the myocardium (heart muscle). By inhibiting phosphodiesterase, Hawthorn's *flavans* have a favorable effect on the myocardium's calcium metabolism, thereby increasing its contractile power and promoting its normal rhythm.

USES
This compound is a **restorative & nutritive tonic for the heart** specifically, and the circulatory vessels in general. Although not a specific remedy for any one heart condition, it is still very much recommended as supportive therapy in any functional derangement of the heart such as: **angina, valvular deficiency** (with or without enlargement), **endo-myocarditis** & **pericarditis, tachycardia, "rheumatic heart," cardiac neuralgia, palpitation, "heart weakness"** & associated neurasthenia. It also serves well as adjunct therapy in the treatment of hypertension.

DOSE
Three times per day take 30 to 40 drops in water. Take last dose of the day just before bedtime.

CAUTIONS
Heart disease and hypertension can be very serious health problems and should be treated under the guidance of a qualified health care practitioner.

Hawthorn can potentiate the *cardiac glycoside* action of Digitalis (or other related drugs like Digitoxin, Digoxin, Gitalin, etc.). Therefore, those who take these drugs while taking Hawthorn should have their Digitalis medication monitored by a physician.

CHILDREN'S COMPOUND
Tonic for Babies & Small Children

A blend of the liquid extracts of:
★ **Chamomile flower** (Matricaria chamomilla)	20%
★ **Lemon Balm leaf & flower** (Melissa off.)	18%
★ **Catnip leaf & flower** (Nepeta cataria)	18%
● **Fennel seed** (Foeniculum vulgare)	14%
Vegetable Glycerine, USP	30%

★ Fresh ● Dried

ACTION
The four herbs in this compound are classic folk remedies that have proven themselves to be reliable and safe in the home health care of babies and small children. The collective actions of these herbs are: antibacterial & antiviral, anti-inflammatory, carminative (expel gas), antispasmodic, gently sedative, mildly astringent, soothingly expectorant, and best of all, they taste good.

USES
Although not a panacea, this compound can be helpful in most ordinary health problems of children. It is indicated in: **feverish conditions** (**colds, flu, coughs**, etc.); **diarrhea, upset tummy** and **colic**; and as a gentle sedative for the fretting and peevishness associated with **teething** or other irritating or **nervous conditions**. It can also help in treating **infant jaundice**.

DOSE
Serving size is 1 drop per 4 pounds of child's body weight (e.g. 10 drops for a 40 pound child).

Give two to five servings per day mixed in water or juice.

For feverish conditions, drops are best taken in hot water in order to induce a sweat — otherwise take with room-temperature water.

ADJUNCT THERAPY
The addition of 5 to 15 drops of ECHINACEA EXTRACT or ECHINACEA GLYCERITE to each dose of the above is recommended in any infection, especially if there is fever.

CAUTIONS
There are no known contraindications to this compound, although one must be very careful not to let the child get chilled if sweating.

This compound is not a substitute for professional health care. If fever, pain or other symptoms are severe or persistent, promptly seek qualified healthcare.

COLLINSONIA • HORSE CHESTNUT COMPOUND
Restorative Venous Tonic

A blend of the liquid extracts of:
★ **Collinsonia, lf., flr. & rhizome** (Collinsonia canadensis) 24%
★ **Horse Chestnut seed** (Aesculus hippocastanus) 24%
• **Butcher's Broom rhizome** (Ruscus aculeatus) 24%
★ **Rosemary flowering branches** (Rosmarinus off.) 18%
• **Prickly Ash bark** (Xanthoxylum clava-herculis) 10%
★ Fresh • Dried

ACTION
Improves tone of venous endothelium, and reduces vascular fragility. Inhibits perivascular edema by reducing permeability of venous walls, and facilitates reabsorbtion of edematous fluids back into the capillaries. Platelet anti-aggregate constituents assist in preventing venous thrombosis.

USES
Venous stasis and atony of venous circulation: **varicose veins**, **hematomas**, **phlebitis**, and **chronically incompetent veins**; cramps, heaviness & fatigue in the legs, particularly at the end of the day; painful veins during menstruation; **hemorrhoids** (piles); prevention and treatment of **thrombosis** & **thrombophlebitis**; **edematous swelling** of bruises, fractures, strokes & brain trauma; **lymphoedema** & **lymphostasis**; **cold hands** & **feet**.

DOSE
Preventative tonic: One or two times per day take 20 to 30 drops in water.

Restorative tonic for chronic conditions: Three times per day take 30 to 40 drops in water.

Acute: Three to five times per day take 40 to 50 drops in water.

Note: Do not take more than 150 drops within 24 hours. During pregnancy, or for continued use, take the *restorative tonic* dose 6 days per week, for 6 weeks; then skip a week (take no drops); then repeat the same cycle again.

Topical: Apply gently over troubled area (varicose veins, bruises, hematomas, etc.). Can be used undiluted in most cases, but should be diluted (50 drops per ounce of water) for sensitive areas and hemorrhoids. Apply around broken skin and varicose ulcers but not directly to them — it is best to use HERBAL SALVE here.

ADJUNCT THERAPY

THUJA • GOTU KOLA COMPOUND is helpful as a restorative to venous & capillary connective tissues. Take 40 drops 2 or 3 times per day.

HERBAL LINIMENT can be applied to varicose veins to improve local circulation and enhance action of above compounds. Apply as described above under "Topical."

For associated pigmentation, eczema & skin ulcers apply HERBAL SALVE.

ECHINACEA EXTRACT should be used during any inflammatory stage (phlebitis, "burning" veins or hemorrhoids, etc.). Take 30 to 40 drops 3 to 5 times per day.

Physiotherapy for legs: External elastic support (stockings or bandages) can often ameliorate symptoms and may impede progression of venous deterioration. This can be especially important in pregnancy. Here the woman should put on support stockings before she first stands on arising.

To relieve edema and other complications, the legs should be elevated above heart level several times during the day. For sleeping, the foot of the bed should be raised about 2 inches. Avoid standing or sitting for more than one hour at a time.

Obesity is a contributory cause of varicose veins — lose weight if need be.

CAUTIONS

Because of the Horse Chestnut in this compound, seek expert medical advice before taking during pregnancy or nursing, or in cases of liver or kidney diseases.

Although venous disease can often be mild and self-limiting, some cases can become serious health problems and, with the associated danger of pulmonary embolism, can be a threat to life. It is therefore important that venous disease be treated by a qualified healthcare practitioner.

CORN SILK • PLANTAIN COMPOUND

Urinary Incontinence Remedy

A blend of the liquid extracts of:

★ **Corn Silk** [stigma & style] (Zea mays)   25%
★ **Plantain leaf** (Plantago lanceolata)   25%
★ **St. John's Wort flower & bud** (Hypericum perf.)   25%
★ **Thuja leaf** (Thuja occidentalis)   15%
• **Arnica flower** (Arnica montana)   10%

★ Fresh   • Dried

ACTION

Soothing to inflamed and irritated tissues of the lower urinary tract. Helps restore natural elasticity to flaccid tissue of the urinary bladder, urethra & ureter. Favorably augments neurological innervation to over-relaxed urinary sphincters and thereby helps restore their natural tone.

USES

Indicated in **urinary weakness & incontinence** of the aged, and "**bed wetting**" of children.

DOSE

Adults: Three times per day take 30 to 40 drops in water.

Children: Adjust above adult doses according to child's body weight (see Clark's Rule, pg. 128).

Continued use for chronic conditions: Take drops 2 times per day, 6 days per week, for several weeks to several months. Two to four, or even six months' use may be needed for full results.

ADJUNCT THERAPY

In cases associated with painful or burning urination, take drops with URINARY TEA BLEND.

CAUTIONS

Urinary incontinence is sometimes associated with urinary tract infections which can lead to serious medical consequences. If symptoms persist for more than a few days, and especially if there is pain or fever, promptly seek qualified healthcare.

DANDELION • MILK THISTLE COMPOUND
Liver & Gall Bladder Tonic

A blend of the liquid extracts of:

★ **Dandelion root, leaf & flower** (Taraxacum off.)   20%
● **Oregon Grape root** (Berberis aquifolium)   20%
● **Milk Thistle mature seed** (Silybum marianum)   20%
● **Artichoke leaf** (Cynara scolymus)   16%
★ **Beet leaf** (Beta vulgaris)   16%
● **Fennel seed** (Foeniculum vulgare)   8%

★ Fresh   ● Dried

ACTION
This compound is a restorative & protective tonic for the liver, and is cleansing to both the liver and gall bladder.

USES
Can be used as an occasional maintenance tonic, or to cleanse and strengthen after illness or abuse, or in the treatment of hepatic & biliary illness (acute or chronic). Indicated in **hepatic torpor, hepatitis, jaundice, sluggish bile** and **gallstones**, and as adjunct therapy in **chronic constipation**. Also used for post-surgical treatment in cases of **cholecystectomy** (gall bladder removal).

DOSE
Tonic: Mix 30 to 40 drops in water and take after meals.

Acute or severe chronic: Mix 30 to 40 drops in water and take after meals. If nausea or hepatic pain results (which is rare) lower the number of drops and take with *Fennel seed tea*.

CAUTIONS
If pain or irritation of the liver or gall bladder persists, and especially if there is high or persistent fever or prolonged nausea and vomiting, promptly seek qualified healthcare.

DEVIL'S CLUB • JAMBUL COMPOUND
Sugar Metabolism Tonic

A blend of the liquid extracts of:
- **Devil's Club root bark** (Oplopanax horridum)   30%
- **Jambul seed** (Syzygium jambolanum)   20%
- ★ **Blueberry leaf** (Vaccinum ovatum)   18%
- **Bean pod** [without beans] (Phaseolus vulgaris)   18%
- ★ **Dandelion root, leaf & flower** (Taraxacum off.)   14%

★ Fresh   • Dried

ACTION & USES
A tonic for restoring and maintaining sugar metabolism equilibrium. Indicated in both **hypoglycemia**, and **hyperglycemia** (**diabetes mellitus**). With regular use of this compound, some diabetics have been able to lower their insulin dosage.*

DOSE
Mix 30 to 45 drops in water and take one-half hour *before* meals.

ADJUNCT THERAPY
GTF CHROMIUM and ZINC supplements can sometimes prove helpful in sugar metabolism problems.

CAUTIONS
This compound is not a substitute for insulin therapy. Diabetics are encouraged to follow the insulin therapy prescribed by their physician.

* Diabetics who take this compound while on insulin therapy should monitor their blood sugar very regularly in case their insulin needs should change and an adjustment of insulin dosage is necessary.

ECHINACEA • BAPTISIA COMPOUND
Immune System Tonic

A blend of the liquid extracts of:
★ **Echinacea root, leaf & flower** (Echinacea purp.) 25%
★ **Wild Indigo root** (Baptisia tinctoria) 25%
★ **Thuja leaf** (Thuja occidentalis) 20%
● **Boneset leaf & flower** (Eupatorium perf.) 20%
● **Prickly Ash bark** (Xanthoxylum clava-herculis) 10%
★ Fresh ● Dried

ACTION
The herbs in this compound have been shown to augment the body's natural ability to resist disease by strengthening and potentiating the immune system. This includes a cortisone-like activity, anti-tumor activity, and increased production and activity of interferon, macrophages, properdin, fibroblasts, T-lymphocytes (killer T-cells), and lymphokines.

USES
Indicated in any condition associated with a **weak or compromised immune system**. Especially indicated for those whose "resistance is down" and are therefore prone to every "bug" that comes around, and those who are plagued by recurring infections, or are slow to heal.

Specific as immuno-supportive therapy in treatment of all **infections** (bacterial, viral & fungal), **chronic inflammatory diseases** (e.g., arthritis), **allergies**, **AIDS**, and **cancer**.

DOSE
Acute: Two to five times per day take 30 to 40 drops in water.

Continued use in chronic conditions: Two or three times per day take 20 to 40 drops in water. Take drops 6 days per week, for 6 weeks; then skip a week (take no drops); then repeat the same cycle. One to three months' use may be necessary for full results.

ADJUNCT THERAPY
In persistent or severe cases, add 30 to 40 drops of Echinacea Extract to the above doses.

CAUTIONS
This compound is not a substitute for qualified healthcare. If you have a condition which requires medical attention you should promptly seek qualified healthcare. This is especially true in cases of AIDS and cancer, or any condition involving high or persistent fever or pain.

ECHINACEA • GOLDENSEAL COMPOUND
Colds & Flu Remedy

A blend of the liquid extracts of:

★ **Echinacea root** (Echinacea purpurea) — 12.50%
● **Goldenseal rhizome & roots** (Hydrastis canadensis) — 12.50%
● **Osha root** (Ligusticum porteri) — 12.50%
★ **Spilanthes flowering herb & root** (Spilanthes ole.) — 12.50%
● **Yerba Santa leaf** (Eriodictyon californicum) — 12.50%
● **Horseradish root** (Cochlearia armoracia) — 12.50%
● **Elder flower** (Sambucus canadensis) — 6.25%
● **Yarrow flower** (Achillea millefolium) — 6.25%
★ **Watercress herb** (Nasturtium officinale) — 6.25%
★ **Wild Indigo root** (Baptisia tinctoria) — 6.25%

★ Fresh   ● Dried

ACTION & USES

For the treatment of **colds** and **flu** — especially when aggravated by congestive nasal and respiratory symptoms.

Can also be used as a strengthening, preventative tonic for those who catch colds and flu easily.

DOSE

Acute: Three to five times per day take 30 to 40 drops in water or DIAPHORETIC TEA. If this treatment is started at the very first sign of symptoms, the cold or flu can usually be aborted within 12 to 24 hours. In persistent cases, adding 30 to 40 drops of ECHINACEA EXTRACT to the above doses is often helpful.

Preventative Tonic: Mix 30 to 40 drops in water and take 3 times per day; especially indicated during the change of seasons or anytime an impending flu or cold is suspected.

ADJUNCT THERAPY

DIAPHORETIC ("SWEATING") TEA: Made with equal parts Elder flowers, Yarrow flowers, and Peppermint leaves. Pour 16 ounces of boiling water over 2 heaping tablespoons of tea blend, cover & let steep for 20 minutes, strain, and drink while still hot. **Note:** Keep body & feet warm and covered, and do not go into the cold for at least one hour after drinking this tea.

CAUTIONS

Sometimes colds and flu can turn into pneumonia, strep throat, ear infections, or other serious complications — be on the lookout for this. In cases of high or persistent fever, or other serious symptoms, promptly seek qualified healthcare.

ELEUTHERO • LICORICE COMPOUND
Restorative Adrenal Gland Tonic

A blend of the liquid extracts of:
- **Siberian Ginseng root** (Eleutherococcus sent.)   25%
- **Licorice root** (Glycyrrhiza glabra)   25%
- ★ **Oat "milky" seed** (Avena sativa)   20%
- **Jamaican Sarsaparilla root** (Smilax ornata)   20%
- **Prickly Ash bark** (Xanthoxylum clava-herculis)   10%

★ Fresh   • Dried

ACTION
Siberian Ginseng, Licorice & Sarsaparilla contain natural *phytosterols* (plant steroids) which are chemically similar to the steroid hormones produced by the adrenal glands. Many herbalists believe these herbs are supportive or restorative to the adrenals, and there is some scientific evidence to support this.

USES
Exhaustion and diminished function of the adrenal glands caused by frequent or prolonged stress. This includes the physical and mental stresses associated with injury, illness, prolonged pain, overwork or severe exertion, mental strain, worry and anxiety. Especially indicated when "low energy" and lack of vitality are associated with mild adrenal hypofunction (under-activity).

May be helpful as supportive therapy when treating Addison's Disease* (chronic adrenocortical insufficiency) and other adrenal-deficient maladies manifesting as anemia, general languor and debility, low blood pressure, or feeble heart action.

DOSE
Maintenance Tonic: Two times per day take 30 to 40 drops in water.

Restorative Tonic: Three times per day take 30 to 40 drops in water. One to three months' use may be needed for full results.

CAUTIONS
* Addison's Disease and other diseases of the adrenal glands can be very injurious or even fatal if not treated properly. This compound is not a substitute for qualified healthcare in such cases.

Although this compound is unlikely to do harm, its use in hyperadrenal conditions is contraindicated. This is especially true in Cushing's syndrome (excess of cortisol hormone) and Conn's syndrome (excess of aldosterone).

The extra energy experienced from taking this compound may create sleeplessness. If this happens decrease dosage or do not take drops in the evening.

ERIGERON • CINNAMON COMPOUND
Hemostatic & Anti-Hemorrhagic Remedy

A blend of essential oils & alcohol:
Ceylon Cinnamon Bark oil (Cinnamomum zeylanicum) 6.25%
Erigeron flowering herb oil (Erigeron canadensis)   6.25%
Grain Alcohol, USP   87.50%

This is the original formula developed by the famous Eclectic physician, Finley Ellingwood, M.D., which he stated was "an extemporaneous prescription, which is (my) first resort in passive hemorrhage."

ACTION & USES
Dr. Ellingwood states in his American Materia Medica, Therapeutics & Pharmacognosy, that Cinnamon "...is a hæmostatic of much power and positively reliable in all passive hemorrhages," and that "...it acts in perfect harmony with Erigeron..." He goes on to say that it "...works to a better advantage in **hemorrhage due to atonic conditions** of the non-gravid womb, or where there is muscular relaxation, or a general flaccid state of the womb after delivery."

"It certainly **restores tone to the uterine muscular structure** and induces tonic contraction. In some cases, during labor, it promotes the normal labor pains and materially increases uterine contraction, and **prevents postpartum hemorrhage**."

Dr. Ellingwood used his compound "...in all the uterine conditions named above, in extreme **pulmonary hemorrhage**, persistent **hæmoptysis**, and in **gastric and intestinal hemorrhages** of alcoholics. In all forms of hæmaturia, especially in renal tuberculosis, and in habitual **nasal hemorrhage**, in many cases, a single dose accomplishes the object."

DOSE
Dr. Ellingwood states, "It is not advisable to combine it with the usual astringents, as ergot, geranium or epilobium..."

For dosage he states, "Ten to 30 drops on sugar, or dropped at once on water, will control nearly every controllable passive hemorrhage."

CAUTIONS
Dr. Ellingwood states, "It is somewhat of an irritant to the stomach, especially if full doses be given for a protracted period."

Hemorrhage can be life-threatening. In any case of hemorrhaging, immediately seek qualified healthcare!

EYEBRIGHT • NETTLE COMPOUND
Hayfever & Allergy Remedy

A blend of the liquid extracts of:
- ★ **Eyebright flowering herb** (Euphrasia officinalis) 34%
- **Goldenseal rhizome & roots** (Hydrastis canadensis) 20%
- **Horseradish root** (Cochlearia armoracia) 18%
- **Nettle mature seed** (Urtica dioica) 14%
- **Yarrow flower** (Achillea millefolium) 14%

★ Fresh   • Dried

ACTION
Astringent, anti-inflammatory, and decongestant to the membranes of the eyes, nose & sinuses, and the throat and upper respiratory tract.

USES
Specific for symptomatic relief of **hayfever & other allergies** which manifest as **acute catarrhal inflammation of the ocular**, **nasal**, **upper respiratory & throat membranes**, with sneezing, profuse watery secretion, or abundant flow of acrid mucous.

DOSE
Acute: Three to five times per day take 30 to 40 drops in water.

Chronic: Two to three times per day take 30 to 40 drops in water.

ADJUNCT THERAPY
Echinacea • Baptisia Compound may be helpful in certain persistent allergy conditions associated with a weakened immune system.

CAUTIONS
Although this compound can often give symptomatic relief, it is not a cure for hayfever and other allergies.

In certain cases of severe allergic reaction, life-threatening anaphylactic shock can ensue. In such a case seek qualified emergency medical care at once!

FEVERFEW • LAVENDER COMPOUND
Headache & Migraine Remedy

A blend of the liquid extracts of :
- **Feverfew leaf & flower** (Tanacetum parthenium)   40%
- **Meadowsweet leaf & flower** (Spiræa ulmaria)   30%
- ★ **Periwinkle flowering tips** (Vinca major)   20%
- **Lavender flower** (Lavandula vera)   10%

★ Fresh   • Dried

ACTION
Medical researchers have proven that the daily intake of Feverfew can successfully decrease the frequency of migraine attacks or cause them to be less painful, or both. *(British Medical Journal*, Vol. 291, Aug. 1985)

USES
This compound is often effective in relieving many kinds of headaches, including: the occasional **simple headache**, **migraines** (acute and chronic), and **cluster headaches**.

Note: There are many types of headaches that can be caused by many different things (tension & worry, toxemia, pH imbalance, etc.). Therefore, in using this compound one should ideally also remove the root cause of the headache.

DOSE
The sooner this compound is used, the better it will work. Therefore, begin using at the very first sign of a headache.

Acute: Take an initial dose of 30 to 40 drops mixed in water. Often this one dose is all that is needed. If headache remains or returns, take 20 to 30 more drops, depending upon severity. This can be done up to 5 times per day.

Chronic Migraines: For extended therapy against chronic migraines, two to three times per day take 20 to 40 drops in water. This can take from 4 to 6 weeks before full results are obtained.

CAUTIONS
Sometimes headaches can be associated with severe disease (e.g., brain tumors, blood clots, etc.). Headaches that are severe, long lasting, or frequently recurring may indicate more serious illness and the need to seek the help of a qualified healthcare practitioner.

FRIAR'S BALSAM
An Antiseptic Vulnerary & A Stimulating Expectorant

A blend of the liquid extracts of:
- **Siam Benzoin resin** (Styrax tonkinensis)   47%
- ◆ **Storax balsam** (Liquidambar orientalis)   17%
- ◆ **Balsam of Tolu** (Toluifera balsamum)   17%
- ◆ **Balsam of Peru** (Toluifera pareiræ)   9%
- **Aloe leaf latex** (Aloe barbadensis)   4%
- **Myrrh tears** (Commiphora abyssinica)   4%
- **Angelica root** (Angelica archangelica)   2%

   ● Dried   ◆ Liquid Exudate

Through its 600-year history, *Friar's Balsam* has been known by such names as *Balsamum Traumaticum, Balsamic Tincture, Jesuits' Drops, Jerusalem Drops,* and *Wound, Swedish, Turlington's, Persian, Wade's, St. Victor's,* and *Commander's Balsam.*

ACTION & USES
Can be used as an antiseptic and protectant to minor **cuts & abrasions, chapped skin & lips, cracked nipples, small fissures** of skin & anus, **bedsores, indolent ulcers, herpes simplex**, and **gingivitis**. Can relieve **itching of chilblains, eczema,** and **urticaria**.

Can be taken internally and/or inhaled with steam vapor as a stimulating expectorant in **old coughs & catarrhs, laryngitis**, **acute & chronic bronchitis,** and **asthma**.

DOSE
Topical: Lesion should be cleaned and dried, and then covered with the balsam, over which should be laid fresh cotton gauze, extending well beyond the lesion. This application may be painful at first, and should be changed daily, taking care to remove any dead tissue that is loose.

Internal: Two to four times per day take 25 to 35 drops in water. To make a soothing syrup for throat or bronchial affections, mix drops in a spoonful of honey, maple syrup or malt syrup.

Inhalant: Mix one or two or three dropperfulls of the balsam into a pint of hot, steaming (not boiling) water and then breathe the vapors in deeply.

CAUTIONS
Occasionally skin irritation may result from topical use — avoid use on individuals with allergic skin diseases. If irritation does appear, discontinue use and the it will soon subside.

When applied to broken skin, undiluted extract may tend to sting. To avoid this, balsam can be diluted with a 50/50 mixture of water & glycerin. Discontinue use if irritation persists.

Some of the maladies listed above can be serious health threats if not treated properly by a qualified healthcare practitioner.

GINGER • CAYENNE COMPOUND
Warming, Circulation Enhancing Tonic

A blend of the liquid extracts of:
★ **Ginkgo leaf** (Ginkgo biloba)   25%
● **Siberian Ginseng root** (Eleutherococcus senticosus)   25%
★ **Rosemary flowering branches** (Rosmarinus officinalis) 20%
● **Ginger rhizome** (Zingiber officinale)   16%
● **Prickly Ash bark** (Xanthoxylum clava-herculis)   10%
● **Cayenne pepper** (Capsicum annuum var. frutescens) 1:4   4%

★ Fresh   ● Dried

ACTION
Enhances the general circulation of the blood and warms the extremities; promotes venous and capillary integrity.

USES
Indicated in overall **poor circulation**, especially when associated with pallor & coldness of the extremities (**cold hands & feet**). Also may be useful as adjunct therapy in the treatment of Raynaud's disease, intermittent claudication, varicose veins, hemorrhoids, & arteriosclerosis.

DOSE
Two to four times per day take 20 to 40 drops in water. Best taken upon arising and between meals.

A stimulating "hot toddy" which warms the innards and defrosts the body from the cold winds of winter can be made by mixing drops into hot apple juice.

ADJUNCT THERAPY
HERBAL LINIMENT can be massaged into cold hands & feet to invigorate the skin and local circulation.

For Raynaud's disease massage LOBELIA • SKUNK CABBAGE COMPOUND ("Antispasmodic Tincture") into painful area(s) to relieve spasm of small arteries & arterioles.

CAUTIONS
Do not take when there is fever or active inflammation in the body; especially contraindicated in acute, inflammatory venous diseases associated with burning, redness & pain, as in flare-ups of phlebitis, varicose veins, hemorrhoids, etc.

GINSENG • SARSAPARILLA COMPOUND

Sexual Tonic for Men

A blend of the liquid extracts of:
- **Jamaican Sarsaparilla root** (Smilax ornata)   25%
- **Ginseng root** (Panax ginseng)   25%
- **Saw Palmetto berry** (Serenoa serrulata)   20%
- ★ **Oat "milky" seed** (Avena sativa)   20%
- **Cardamon seed & pod** (Elettaria cardamomum)   10%

★ Fresh   • Dried

ACTION
This compound is an adaptogenic tonic with an emphasis on the sexual energy enhancing properties of adaptogens. Its overall action is to nourish & tone the male sexual glands and to enhance their healthy production of sexual hormones.

USES
Can be used as a maintenance tonic to maintain good sexual health, and as a restorative tonic in cases of **sexual weakness**. Specifically indicated in cases of **sexual exhaustion, debility** & **neurasthenia**, and is especially indicated for **male sexual impotence**.

DOSE
Maintenance Tonic: Two or three times per day take 30 to 40 drops in water.

Restorative Tonic: Three or four times per day take 40 to 50 drops in water.

CAUTIONS
The extra energy experienced from taking this formula may cause sleeplessness in some men. If this happens do not take drops in the evening.

There are no known contraindications to this compound. However, sexual dysfunction may indicate more serious medical problems which should be diagnosed & treated by a qualified healthcare practitioner.

GOLDENROD • HORSETAIL COMPOUND
Urinary Tract Tonic

A blend of the liquid extracts of:

★ **Goldenrod flowering tips** (Solidago canadensis)	22.5%
★ **Corn Silk** [stigma & style] (Zea mays)	22.5%
★ **Horsetail herb** (Equisetum arvense)	22.5%
★ **Pipsissewa leaf** (Chimaphila umbellata)	22.5%
• **Juniper berry** (Juniperus communis)	10.0%

★ Fresh   • Dried

ACTION
Gently cleansing, anti-inflammatory, and disinfectant to the entire urinary system, and a restorative tonic for the rejuvenation and strengthening of the urinary tissue.

USES
A mild **diuretic**. Very soothing in "**scalding urine**" and other irritations of the urinary tract. Supportive in the treatment of **inflammation** & **infection** of the kidneys, bladder and urinary ducts (**nephritis, cystitis, urethritis**, etc.).

DOSE
Acute: Three to five times per day take 30 to 40 drops in water or in URINARY TEA BLEND.

Tonic & Chronic: Two or three times per day take 20 to 40 drops in water or in URINARY TEA BLEND.

ADJUNCT THERAPY
For infection & inflammation of the urinary tract add 20 to 40 drops of ECHINACEA EXTRACT to each dose of the above.

CAUTIONS
Urinary infections can sometimes lead to serious medical consequences. If urinary symptoms persist for more than a few days, and especially if there is fever, promptly seek qualified healthcare.

GOTU KOLA • GINKGO COMPOUND
Brain & Memory Tonic

A blend of the liquid extracts of:
- ★ **Gotu Kola herb & root** (Centella asiatica)   25%
- ★ **Ginkgo leaf** (Ginkgo biloba)   25%
- ★ **Passionflower flowering tips** (Passiflora inc. & edu.)   15%
- ★ **Skullcap flowering herb** (Scutellaria lateriflora)   15%
- • **Calamus rhizome** (Acorus calamus)   10%
- ★ **Rosemary flowering branches** (Rosmarinus off.)   10%

★ Fresh   • Dried

ACTION
Ginkgo: Pharmaceutical studies show that Ginkgo leaf can significantly improve the overall metabolism of the brain by enhancing cerebral circulation, increasing ATP production (energy production) in the brain cells, and increasing oxygen supply to the brain while facilitating the elimination of lactic acid, lactates and other metabolic waste products.

Gotu Kola & Calamus: Both of these herbs have been used in combination for hundreds of years in East Indian Ayurvedic Medicine as rejuvenating tonics for the brain and nervous system.

USES
Indicated in **mental fatigue** from studying and other memory work; **failing memory** of old age, **Alzheimer's Disease** & other dementias; as an aid in **recovery from strokes**; and to enhance meditation or mental work.

DOSE
Two to four times per day take 30 to 40 drops in water.

CAUTIONS
This compound is not a substitute for qualified health care in injuries or diseases of the brain. If pathological symptoms are present promptly seek qualified healthcare.

GRINDELIA • SASSAFRAS COMPOUND

Poison Oak, Ivy & Sumac Remedy

A blend of the liquid extracts of:
- **Sassafras root bark** (Sassafras officinale) 50%
- **Grindelia flower & leaf** (Grindelia robusta) 50%
  Menthol Crystals, USP (3.33% w/v)
  - Dried

ACTION & USES

A specific for **allergic contact dermatitis** associated with the plants **Poison Oak, Poison Ivy**, and **Poison Sumac**. Helps relieve the **itching** and can prevent or lessen the occurence of **blisters**. When first applied there is an overall soothing feeling and relief of the itching. Continued use can minimize the intensity and spread of the dermatitis and speed up the healing process.

DOSE

Preparation: As soon as possible wash the exposed areas with hot soapy water in such a way that the soapy water drips immediately off the body and does not drip or flow down and contaminate unexposed areas. Rinse thoroughly any areas that have been exposed to the soapy water.

Topical: Apply to any areas that show signs of itching, irritation or blisters.

Internal: In severe cases additional relief can sometimes be gained by internal use of this compound. Three to five times per day take 30 to 40 drops in water.

CAUTIONS

In cases of severe irritation and/or broken skin, topical application of this compound can sometimes be painful for some individuals. Therefore, at first only apply a small amount to a small area and see how it feels. If there is uncomfortable pain, discontinue use or dilute drops in water and reapply. If there is no pain, continue by applying small amounts until the whole area is covered.

Rarely, certain highly sensitive individuals may have a severe reaction to Poison Oak, Ivy or Sumac which can lead to impaired breathing. If this situation arises or is suspected, immediately seek emergency medical care.

HELONIAS • VIBURNUM COMPOUND

Gynecological Tonic for Women

A blend of the liquid extracts of:
- **Helonias (False Unicorn) rhizome** (Chamælirium lut.)   25%
- **Squaw Vine herb** (Mitchella repens)   25%
- **Cramp Bark** (Viburnum opulus)   20%
- **Blue Cohosh rhizome & roots** (Caulophyllum thal.)   20%
- **Ginger rhizome** (Zingiber officinale)   10%
  - Dried

ACTION & USES

Favorably affects the general health of the uterus and ovaries (and to a milder degree the bladder), and helps maintain their balanced function and structure.

Uterine weakness & atony: helps maintain healthy tone and posture of uterus and bladder and prevents or restores uterine prolapse, malposition or subinvolution. **Menstrual problems:** helps prevent or relieve amenorrhea, dysmenorrhea, menorrhagia and metrorrhagia. **Prenatal tonic:** quiets uneasiness, nausea & erratic pains during pregnancy; diminishes likelihood of premature birth or miscarriage; and prepares for a smoother easier birth. **Postpartum tonic:** helps tone uterus back to a healthy posture, relieves afterpains, and diminishes excessive lochia. **Puberty:** facilitates physical transition into womanhood and in some cases can help to minimize acne. **Menopause:** facilitates a smooth sexual transition and relieves nervousness and hot flashes. **Infertility:** may restore fertility in cases of metabolic malfunction, but not if there are severe structural abnormalities.

Note: For chronic problems this compound works best taken over a longer period of time (1 to 3 months).

DOSE

Restorative Tonic: Two or three times per day take 30 to 40 drops in water or in RASPBERRY LEAF TEA. As with many tonics, full results may take 1 to 3 months.

Prenatal Tonic: Two or three times per day take 30 to 40 drops in water or in RASPBERRY LEAF TEA throughout last trimester. With difficult pregnancies or history of premature birth or miscarriage, use as a tonic may be indicated throughout entire pregnancy.

Acute: Three to five times per day take 30 to 40 drops in water.

CAUTIONS

In any gynecological problem associated with severe pain or bleeding, with high or persistent fever, or other serious symptoms, promptly seek qualified healthcare.

HERBAL LINIMENT
Warming Embrocation

A blend of the liquid extracts of:
* ★ **St. John's Wort flower & bud** (Hypericum perf.) — 15%
* ● **Arnica flower** (Arnica montana) — 15%
* ★ **Melilot flowering tips** [fermented] (Melilotus off.) — 14%
* ● **Wormwood leaf & flower** (Artemisia absinthium) — 14%
* ★ **Rue tops with immature fruit** (Ruta graveolens) — 14%
* ● **Yarrow flower** (Achillea millefolium) — 14%
* ● **Cayenne pepper** (Capsicum annuum var. frut.) 1:4 — 14%

★ Fresh   ● Dried

ACTION
Warming, stimulating counterirritant action enhances local circulation and promotes capillary integrity; anticoagulant.

USES
To ease general **pain & stiffness in joints & muscles** due to aging, arthritis, rheumatism, or overwork, and to treat **sprained joints** and **strained ligaments & tendons**. Can also be applied to **contusions, bruises & hematomas**; **varicose veins, tired heavy legs** & **cold hands & feet**; **insect bites & stings**; and **frostbite**.

DOSE
Two to four times per day rub liberal amounts of liniment into troubled area until well absorbed.

For more intense treatment, moisten gauze with liniment, apply to troubled area, cover with plastic, and tape into place. Leave in place for 4 to 8 hours, then remove and wash area with warm soapy water.

CAUTIONS
Avoid getting liniment into broken skin, mucous membranes or the eyes. If treated area becomes excessively hot, reddened or irritated, or if a rash appears, discontinue use and wash area with warm soapy water to remove any remaining liniment. If liniment gets into the eyes, flush with liberal amounts of cool water.

The health problems listed above can sometimes be serious health problems. Therefore, anyone suffering from any of these maladies should be treated by a qualified healthcare practitioner.

HERBAL SALVE
Soothing Emollient Vulnerary

- **Comfrey root** (Symphytum officinale)
- ★ **St. John's Wort flower & bud** (Hypericum perforatum)
- **Calendula flower** (Calendula officinalis)
- **Plantain leaf** (Plantago lanceolata)
- **Chickweed herb** (Stellaria media)
- **Mullein leaf** (Verbascum thapsus)

Extracted & concentrated into a base of:
Olive Oil, Bee's Wax & Bee's Propolis
★ Fresh   • Dried

ACTION
This herbal salve is a classic example of a topical *vulnerary,* an agent that promotes the healing of wounds to the skin. Its actions are antiseptic, anti-inflammatory, soothing & analgesic, antipruritic (relieves or prevents itching), and it stimulates the regeneration of aged and damaged tissues and their blood vessels.

USES
Indicated in all cases where the skin or other epithelial tissues are wounded, irritated, inflamed, or aged: **cuts, abrasions**, all types of **burns** (thermal & sun burns, radiation burns, and chemical burns), **frostbite, trauma & bruises, ulcerations & erosions, diaper rash, contact dermatitis, aged & weathered skin, chapped skin & lips, hemorrhoids, irritation or degeneration of labial & vaginal tissues, traumatized eyes**, etc.

DOSE
All wounds should be cleaned and disinfected before applying salve.

Thermal & sun burns should be "cooled down" with cold water or ice packs before applying salve.

Topical: Apply salve to troubled area with a mild rubbing action until salve melts, or smear salve onto sterile gauze and tape to area. Can be applied several times per day according to condition. If gauze sticks to wound, moisten with sterile water or hydrogen peroxide before trying to remove. Salve can be removed from wound with warm water & non-perfumed soap.

Herbal Tampon: For intravaginal application smear salve onto the top two-thirds of a tampon and then insert into vagina. Leave in for 4 to 6 hours (best done while sleeping) and then take at least a 16 hour break before applying a fresh herbal tampon. Before treatment a mild vinegar or herbal douche may be useful. If long-range therapy is indicated use herbal tampon once per day, five days per week, three weeks per month. Do not use during menses.

ADJUNCT THERAPY

THUJA•GOTU KOLA COMPOUND taken internally can assist in the repair and maintenance of healthy connective tissue.

Use ECHINACEA EXTRACT to potentiate the body's immune response to inflammation and infection, and to stimulate granulation of epithelial tissues. Three to five times per day take 30 to 40 drops in water.

CAUTIONS

Depending upon their degree and progression, all of the above maladies can possibly become serious health threats. If redness, irritation, infection, fever, pain, or other adverse symptoms increase or persist, or if foul odor appears, promptly seek qualified medical treatment.

HERBAL STEROL COMPOUND
Energy Enhancing Tonic for Athletes

A blend of the liquid extracts of:
- **Jamaican Sarsaparilla root** (Smilax ornata) 30%
- **Saw Palmetto berry** (Serenoa serrulata) 30%
- **Siberian Ginseng root** (Eleutherococcus sen.) 30%
- ★ **Gotu Kola herb & root** (Centella asiatica) 10%

★ Fresh ● Dried

ACTION
The herbs in this compound contain natural *phytosterols* (plant steroids). The metabolic effects of phytosterols are not as fast-acting or dynamic as synthetic anabolic steroids but, unlike synthetic steroids, they are safe to use and do not have health-threatening side-effects.

Contrary to popular belief, Sarsaparilla root does not contain testosterone. However, Sarsaparilla root has been used in the pharmaceutical industry as the starting material in the manufacture of semi-synthetic testosterone, and is believed by many herbalists (although not proven) to augment the body's natural production of its own testosterone.

USES
This compound can be used in **athletic training & competition** as a safe alternative to synthetic anabolic steroids. It is indicated for both men and women athletes. It is recommended In any situation where the body (or mind) is being trained to perform optimally and is being pushed beyond its normal limits. Facilitates rapid recovery from strenuous physical stress.

DOSE
Three or four times per day take 30 to 50 drops in water. Best taken between meals and a few minutes before physical (or mental) workout.

CAUTIONS
Although this compound is unlikely to do harm, its use in hyperadrenal conditions is contraindicated. This is especially true in Cushing's syndrome (excess of cortisol hormone) and Conn's syndrome (excess of aldosterone).

The extra energy experienced from taking this compound may create sleeplessness. If this happens decrease dosage or do not take drops in the evening.

KHELLA • TURMERIC COMPOUND
Remedy for Chronic Bronchial Asthma

A blend of the liquid extracts of:
- **Khella mature seed** (Ammi visnaga)   30%
- **Skunk Cabbage rhizome & roots** (Dracontium foe.) 20%
- **Grindelia leaf & flower** (Grindelia robusta)   18%
- **Turmeric rhizome** (Curcuma longa)   18%
- **Thyme leaf & flower** (Thymus vulgaris)   14%
  - Dried

ACTION
The actions of the various herbs in this compound overlap to a large degree, but chiefly they are: bronchodilation (Khella), antispasmodic (Skunk Cabbage & Thyme), anti-inflammatory (Turmeric, Grindelia & Thyme), and expectorant (Turmeric, Grindelia & Thyme).

USES
Specific for treating **chronic bronchial asthma**, and **mild asthma attacks**. With continued use this compound can moderate or eliminate chronic symptoms experienced between attacks (**shortness of breath** & **wheezing**), and can lessen the frequency of attacks and diminish their duration and intensity.

DOSE
Palliative tonic between attacks: Two to four times per day take 30 to 40 drops in a little water or, better yet, in strong *Licorice Root Tea*. To facilitate undisturbed sleep take the last dose of the day just before retiring. Continued treatment for several weeks is sometimes needed to achieve best results.

Treating mild attacks: Give 30 to 40 drops in a little water every 1 to 3 hours, depending upon severity of attack and response to treatment. Do not give more than 8 doses in a 24 hour period.

ADJUNCT THERAPY
In *bronchial* asthmas (not cardiac asthmas) associated with irregular heart action and impaired pulmonary circulation, take 30 to 40 drops of CACTUS • HAWTHORN COMPOUND 2 or 3 times per day.

To moderate nervousness or anxiety associated with asthma take 30 to 40 drops of AVENA • SKULLCAP COMPOUND 3 times per day.

Asthma symptoms can sometimes be moderated or eliminated by rubbing undiluted LOBELIA EXTRACT into the upper chest and upper back (between the shoulder blades).

LOBELIA • SKUNK CABBAGE COMPOUND can often be helpful as an adjunct or substitute remedy when the above treatments fail to achieve full results.

Metabolic dysfunction of the liver is often associated with asthma. Therefore, liver restoratives such as DANDELION • MILK THISTLE COMPOUND, may assist in the successful treatment of asthma.

Excellent relief from asthma can often be seen by eliminating from the diet white sugar, white flour, and especially dairy products.

CAUTIONS

The above information does not apply to cardiac asthmas (asthma-like symptoms caused by heart disease).

In *severe* asthmatic attacks the above treatments may help to some degree, but it will probably be necessary to utilize more potent medicine in these cases.

Asthma can often be a serious health problem, and can even be life-threatening. Therefore, anyone suffering from asthma should be treated by a qualified healthcare practitioner.

LAVENDER SPIRITS COMPOUND
Aromatic Carminative & Antinauseant

A blend of the liquid extracts of:
- **Cinnamon bark** (Cinnamomum zeylanicum)   36%
- **Nutmeg seed** (Myristica fragrans)   18%
- **Red Saunders wood** (Pterocarpus santalinus)   18%
- ◆ **Lavender flower** [essential oil] (Lavendula vera)   15%
- **Clove flower bud** (Eugenia caryophyllus)   09%
- ◆ **Rosemary herb** [essential oil] (Rosmarinus officinalis) 04%

● Dried   ◆ Steam-distilled

ACTION
This pleasant tasting compound is a soothing, mildly-warming stimulant to the gastrointestinal mucosa, making it an excellent carminative and antinauseant.

USES
Useful in allaying the **nausea & queasiness** associated with general gastrointestinal maladies such as **dyspepsia**, **colic**, **motion sickness**, **diarrhea**, **morning sickness**, **nervous stomach**, **headache**, **flatulence**, etc.

DOSE
Take 30 to 60 drops in water as needed. Can be taken up to 5 or 6 times per day unless otherwise contraindicated.

CAUTIONS
Because of its warming action on the mucosa, this compound may be contraindicated in cases of severe inflammation or irritation of the gastrointestinal tract. Discontinue use if exacerbation of symptoms occurs.

If nausea or vomiting is severe or persistent, or is associated with pain, bleeding or fever, promptly seek qualified healthcare.

LINDEN • MISTLETOE COMPOUND

High Blood Pressure Remedy

A blend of the liquid extracts of:
- **Hawthorn berry, leaf & flower** (Crataegus oxy.) 25%
- ★ **Olive leaf** (Olea europaea) 25%
- **Linden flower** (Tilia cordata & platyphyllos) 20%
- **Bean pod** [without beans] (Phaseolus vulgaris) 20%
- ★ **Mistletoe herb** (Viscum album) 10%

★ Fresh • Dried

ACTION
Although specific for normalizing high blood pressure, this compound also has a general action as a cardiovascular tonic, and serves as a mild diuretic to remove excess water from the system. For more detail on the action of Hawthorn see CACTUS • HAWTHORN COMPOUND.

USES
Indicated as an aid in treating **essential hypertension** (high blood pressure) and its associated **arteriosclerosis** ("hardening of the arteries"). May help with **headaches**, **dizziness**, **vertigo** & **irritability** associated with hypertension.

DOSE
Three times per day take 30 to 40 drops in a little water. Best taken between meals.

ADJUNCT THERAPY
GOLDENROD • HORSETAIL COMPOUND and/or URINARY TEA BLEND are indicated for their soothing diuretic and restorative actions on the kidneys.

RAW ONIONS contain Prostaglandin A1 which has a hypotensive action.

GARLIC is a time proven remedy for high blood pressure and it contains the natural substance, *ajone,* which is an antithrombotic factor that inhibits the fibrinogen receptors on blood platelets. Eat lots of raw garlic, or, if odor is a problem, take one teaspoon twice a day of GARLIC EXTRACT.

CAUTIONS
Do not take this compound during pregnancy.

High blood pressure can be a very serious, life-threatening disease if left untreated or if treated improperly. It is very important that high blood pressure be monitored and treated under the supervision of a qualified physician.

LOBELIA • SKUNK CABBAGE COMPOUND
Antispasmodic Tincture

A blend of the liquid extracts of:
- **Lobelia herb, & mature seed** (Lobelia inflata)   18%
- **Skunk Cabbage rhizome & roots** (Dracontium foe.) 18%
- ★ **Skullcap flowering herb** (Scutellaria lateriflora)   18%
- **Black Cohosh rhizome & roots** (Cimicifuga rac.)   18%
- **Myrrh tears** (Commiphora abyssinica)   18%
- **Cayenne pepper** (Capsicum annuum var. frutescens) 10%

★ Fresh   • Dried

HISTORY
Antispasmodic Tincture is a tried and true remedy in American traditional herbal medicine. It was made famous by the renowned American herbalist, Jethro Kloss, in his classic American herbal, Back To Eden, which was first published in 1939.

ACTION
This compound is both a strong, relaxing antispasmodic, and a powerful diffusive stimulant. It acts to relieve muscular and visceral tensions in the body while vitalizing & equalizing the neurological force and the circulation of the blood and body fluids.

USES
In Back To Eden Jethro Kloss recommended *Antispasmodic Tincture* for the following conditions: **asthma**, **whooping cough**, **spasmodic croup**, **cramps**, **spasms**, **convulsions**, **epilepsy**, **suspended animation**, **hysteria**, **fainting**, **delirium tremens**, **childbirth**, **hydrophobia**, & **lockjaw**. He also advised: "Apply externally to **any kind of swelling, cramps**; is very beneficial in **rheumatism, lumbago**, etc."

It is my opinion that this compound could possibly be helpful in the treatment of multiple sclerosis or Parkinson's disease.

DOSE
Preventative or restorative tonic: Two to three times per day take 15 to 30 drops in water.*

Acute: Three to five times per day take 20 to 40 drops in water.*

**The following information is given by
Jethro Kloss in his famous herbal, <u>Back To Eden</u>.**
"We have given just a drop or two on the tip of the finger, thrusting the finger into the mouth of a baby in convulsions, and in less time than it takes to write this statement the convulsions have ceased."

"Dr. H. Nowell has poured a teaspoonful of the antispasmodic tincture, full strength, between the clenched teeth of a case of lockjaw and before a second teaspoonful could be poured from the bottle the locked jaws have relaxed."

"... in the case of infants, it should be rubbed well into the neck, chest, and between the shoulders at the same time. Two or three drops of the tincture in a raw state should be placed in the mouth and washed down with teaspoonful doses of warm water and the patient kept warm in bed. In all such cases relief will be experienced in a few minutes, and by repeating the same treatment every one or two hours a cure will soon be effected and the patient brought to a state of convalescence."

CAUTIONS
* Because of the Lobelia in this compound, large and frequent doses may induce nausea or vomiting in some sensitive individuals. If this happens, discontinue use for 1 or 2 days, and then resume use with a lower number of drops. Drops can be adjusted according to tolerance.

This compound is contraindicated for asthenic individuals with low vitality and a weak constitution, and in cases of low blood pressure.

Many of the maladies listed above can often be serious health problems or even life-threatening. Anyone suffering from any of these maladies should be treated by a qualified healthcare practitioner.

LOMATIUM • ST. JOHN'S WORT COMPOUND
Antiviral Remedy

A blend of the liquid extracts of:

★ **Lomatium root** (Lomatium dissectum)		20%
★ **St. John's Wort flower & bud** (Hypericum perf.)		20%
• **Hyssop leaf & flower** (Hyssopus officinalis)		16%
★ **Lemon Balm leaf & flower** (Melissa off.)		16%
★ **Thuja leaf** (Thuja occidentalis)		16%
• **Echinacea mature seed** (Echinacea purpurea)		12%

★ Fresh   • Dried

ACTION
Echinacea helps to potentiate the body's natural production of virus inhibiting interferon, and all of the other herbs have shown direct antiviral activity.

USES
Indicated as adjunct therapy in disease conditions caused by or associated with a virus: **herpes**, **warts**, **Epstein-Barr virus** & **infectious mononucleosis**, **viral meningitis**, **mumps**, **measles**, **encephalitis**, **shingles**, **influenza**, etc.

DOSE
Internal: Two to four times per day take 30 to 40 drops in water. Best taken between meals.

Topical: Apply to the affected area 2 to 5 times per day. For optimal results also take drops internally.

CAUTIONS
Although rare, some sensitive people may develop a skin rash after several days or weeks of ingesting Lomatium root. If this happens, discontinue use of this compound and the rash will soon disappear.

Be aware that viral infections can be serious, and some of the viral diseases listed above can be deadly if not treated promptly under competent medical supervision. If you have a viral infection, and especially if there is fever, promptly seek qualified healthcare.

MADDER • HYDRANGEA COMPOUND
Remedy for Urinary Tract Calculi (Kidney Stones)

A blend of the liquid extracts of:
• **Madder root** (Rubia tinctorum)	35%
• **Hydrangea root** (Hydrangea arborescens)	20%
• **Gravel Root** (Eupatorium purpureum)	20%
• **Burdock mature seed** (Arctium lappa)	15%
• **Horseradish root** (Cochlearia armoracia)	10%

• Dried

ACTION
Although the herbs in this compound are known to be soothing diuretics, their traditional use in preventing and dissolving urinary stones has not, of yet, been explained by modern pharmaceutical science.

USES
Indicated in the treatment of **urinary tract calculi** ("kidney stones") which are located in the kidney, bladder, or ureter. Can also serve as prophylactic therapy to prevent or diminish the tendency to form new stones.

DOSE
Stone Dissolving Therapy: Three times per day mix 50 drops of compound with a pinch of sodium bicarbonate (baking soda) in 8 ounces of water and drink all at once. Best taken between meals. Try this therapy for two months — if there is no success after this time, the therapy is unlikely to be effective.

Stone Prophylactic Therapy: Use the same mixture as above, but with 40 drops of compound, and take just two times per day.

ADJUNCT THERAPY
To sooth the urinary tract drink a pint of URINARY TEA BLEND each day.

For stones that are passing with difficulty it is helpful to dilate the ureter, and also to relieve any inflammatory edema. Mix together 25 drops each of the liquid extracts of KHELLA, HORSE CHESTNUT, CHAMOMILE & PETASITES in 8 ounces of hot water and drink all at once. This can be administered up to 6 times per day. Also apply hot compresses over the kidney area, or soak in a hot bath.

CAUTIONS

Because hematuria (blood in the urine) is often associated with urinary tract stones, the patient should be aware that the red pigments in Madder root can sometimes give a harmless red color to the urine.

Beware of urinary infections which are often associated with stones in the urinary tract.

Urinary tract stones should be properly diagnosed and treated by a qualified healthcare practitioner.

MULLEIN • GARLIC COMPOUND
Herbal Ear Drops

A blend of the olive oil extracts of:
- **Calendula flower** (Calendula officinalis)   30%
- ★ **St. John's Wort flower & bud** (Hypericum perf.)   25%
- ★ **Mullein flower** [no stalk] (Verbascum thapsus)   25%
- ★ **Garlic bulb** (Allium sativum)   20%

★ Fresh   • Dried

ACTION
Inhibits or destroys bacteria or fungus present in the ear canal. Controls inflammation, edema, and itching. Has an analgesic (pain relieving) effect. Softens and disperses accumulated cerumen (earwax). Restorative tonic to the blood vessels in the ear.

USES
Ear infections, congestion & inflammation (otitis media, interna & externa), and associated **earache**; **swimmer's ear**; to **loosen earwax** in preparation for ear cleaning. May also help in certain cases of **tinnitus** ("ringing in the ears"), and **vertigo**.

DOSE
Take care that dropper and bottle mouth do not come into contact with the ear, hands, hair or other sources of contamination.

Roll bottle between the hands for 2 minutes to warm the oil. Do not place cold drops into the ear.

Cleansing: Place 2 or 3 drops into each ear 1 or 2 times per day. Irrigation of ears may be necessary to aid in removal of earwax. Have this done by a physician, or make sure you know how to do it properly.

Acute inflammation & infections: Place 2 or 3 drops into troubled ear 2 or 3 times per day.

ADJUNCT THERAPY
Internal doses of Echinacea Extract are indicated in any ear infection. Three to five times per day drink 30 to 40 drops mixed in a little water.

Hot Onion & Vinegar Poultices applied over the ear can often be very helpful in relieving the congestion & pain associated with ear infections.

GINKGO EXTRACT can enhance the health and function of the blood vessels that supply the ears, and can have a positive influence on diseases of the ear initiated or aggravated by poor blood supply. Two or three times per day drink 30 to 40 drops mixed into a little water. Positive results in chronic degenerative cases can take several months.

CAUTIONS

Orthodox medicine advises not placing liquids in the ear when there is perforation of the eardrum. However, I have seen many cases with perforated eardrum where these herbal ear drops have had excellent results, and I know of no such cases where they have caused a problem. Perhaps they could cause a problem, but that has not been my experience. Please be aware that you are not being advised here to use these ear drops in cases where there is perforated eardrum. That is your decision to make.

Ear infections can sometimes turn into a serious medical problem. Therefore, it is very important to promptly seek qualified medical care in any ear disorder with fever or where redness, pain, or swelling is severe or persists.

NEUTRALIZING CORDIAL
Antacid, Antidiarrhea & Gastro-Intestinal Corrective

A blend of the liquid extracts of:
- **Rhubarb rhizome** (Rheum palmatum)   42%
- **Ceylon Cinnamon inner bark** (Cinnamumum zeylanicum) 33%
- **Goldenseal rhizome & roots** (Hydrastis canadensis) 20%
- ★ **Peppermint Spirits** (Mentha piperita)   5%

In a base of Water, Alcohol, Vegetable Glycerine
& Potassium Carbonate (1.6% w/v).

★ Fresh   • Dried

HISTORY
First developed by Eclectic physicians in the mid-1800s, this remedy was used by American physicians until its use faded (with all herbal medicines) in the 1940s.

ACTION
Agreeable antacid & antidiarrhea. A mild laxative (in large doses). Tones & soothes stomach & intestines and promotes normal action. Stimulates appetite. Carminative (relieves gastro-intestinal pain & flatulence).

USES
Indicated in **fermentative & irritative conditions of stomach & bowels**: Sour stomach, burning belching or vomiting; indigestion & decomposed food; sour, fermented stools; watery, copious diarrhea, irritative diarrhea, diarrhea of undigested food, traveler's diarrhea & dysentery; irritative children's summer diarrhea; muco-enteritis.

In larger doses acts as mild, soothing laxative which is especially indicated for clearing the intestinal tract of sour, decomposed materials.

Neutralizing Cordial's agreeable flavor of peppermint & cinnamon, and its mild action makes it an ideal gastro-intestinal tonic for children in the above conditions.

DOSE
Adults: As a soothing corrective take 30 to 80 drops every 1/2 hour, hour, or 2 hours according to urgency of symptoms. Drops should be well diluted in 4 to 8 ounces of water.

In controlling diarrhea, dose should not exceed more than 80 drops.

As a mild laxative, usually a tablespoonful diluted in a cup of water is sufficient to clear intestines.

Children: Adjust above adult doses according to child's body weight (see Clark's Rule, pg. 128).

ADJUNCT THERAPY
For severe diarrhea add 30 to 40 drops of WILD GERANIUM EXTRACT to above doses.

For extreme lack of stomach or intestinal tone add 30 to 40 drops of PRICKLY ASH EXTRACT or 15 to 25 drops of CAYENNE EXTRACT to above doses.

For sharp colicky pains add 30 to 40 drops of GINGER EXTRACT to above doses.

Children: Adjust above adult doses according to child's body weight (see Clark's Rule, pg. 128).

CAUTIONS
Some of the above conditions may indicate a serious health problem and could require treatment by a qualified healthcare practitioner, especially if there is fever or if symptoms are severe or persistent.

Large or laxative doses should not be used for more than three days, and should be avoided during pregnancy or if there is abdominal pain or diarrhea.

PROPOLIS • ECHINACEA
Herbal Throat Spray
Soothing Antiseptic for Throat & Mouth

A blend of the liquid extracts of:
- **Echinacea root** (Echinacea purpurea)   17%
- **Propolis resin** (Resina propoli)   17%
- **Hyssop leaf & flower** (Hyssopus officinalis)   17%
- **Sage leaf** (Salvia officinalis)   17%
- ★ **St. John's Wort flower & bud** (Hypericum perf.)   17%
- **Vegetable Glycerine, USP**   15%

★ Fresh   • Dried

ACTION
Antiseptic, analgesic & anti-inflammatory to inflamed and infected tissues of mouth, gums, throat & skin. Fights infection, relieves swelling and soothes pain.

USES
Specifically indicated in **infected sore throat**, and enlarged tonsils of **tonsillitis**. Can also be useful in the treatment of **pharyngitis** and **laryngitis**, and to heal sores & ulcerations of the mouth, gums & throat.

This spray can also be useful in the treatment of cuts, scratches, abrasions, sores & ulcerations of the skin.

DOSE
Spray onto affected area(s) 2 or 3 times, and repeat every 1/2 hour, hour or two hours according to severity of symptoms. Be careful not to spray into the eyes.

ADJUNCTS
ECHINACEA EXTRACT can be very helpful in fighting inflammation & infection associated with sore throat & tonsillitis. Three to 6 times per day take 30 to 40 drops in water.

For very sore throat or severe mouth sores, gargle or rinse mouth 3 to 5 times per day with a solution made of 40 drops MYRRH EXTRACT in 2 ounces of water.

For associated swollen lymph glands of throat and/or neck, take 3 to 4 times per day one or more of the following extracts mixed in a little water: ECHINACEA (30 to 40 drops), CEANOTHUS (30 to 40 drops), STILLINGIA (15 to 25 drops) & POKE (5 to 8 drops).

CAUTIONS

Because of its alcohol content, this spray can sting when first applied to open sores, ulcerations or broken skin. However, the pain is short-lived and soon passes.

Sore throat and swollen glands can lead to serious health maladies (especially strep infections). Some of the above conditions may indicate a serious health problem which would require treatment by a qualified healthcare practitioner, especially if symptoms are persistent or there is severe pain or high fever.

PULSATILLA • VITEX COMPOUND
Tonic for Menopausal Women

A blend of the liquid extracts of:
- **Chaste Tree berry** (Vitex agnus-castus)   30%
- **Motherwort leaf & flower** (Leonurus cardiaca)   19%
- **Black Cohosh rhizome & roots** (Cimicifuga rac.) 19%
- ★ **Pulsatilla flowering herb** (Anemone pulsatilla) 16%
- **Licorice root** (Glycyrrhiza glabra)   16%

★ Fresh   • Dried

ACTION
Chaste Tree berries help restore a normal estrogen/progesterone balance by increasing luteinizing hormone production and inhibiting the release of follicle stimulating hormone.

USES
Indicated in relieving the endocrine, somatic, and emotional symptoms associated with **menopause** and **ovarian insufficiency**: fatigue & lassitude; insomnia; nervousness, irritability or depression; heart palpitations; hot flushes & sweating; and related "odd sensations."

DOSE
Two to four times per day take 30 to 40 drops in a little water.

Positive results can take from several days to several weeks.

ADJUNCT THERAPY
If heart palpitations are not relieved add 30 to 40 drops of CACTUS • HAWTHORN COMPOUND to each dose of the above.

CAUTIONS
Certain symptoms blamed on menopause are often not due to menopause at all, and there is a danger of neglecting a specific disorder that could and should be treated. It is therefore important to seek guidance from a qualified healthcare practitioner when experiencing health problems during menopause.

RED CLOVER • STILLINGIA COMPOUND

THE HOXSEY FORMULA
Lymphatic & Glandular Alterative

A blend of the liquid extracts of:
- **Red Clover blossom** (Trifolium pratense)   17%
- **Licorice root** (Glycyrrhiza glabra)   17%
- **Buckthorn bark** [aged 1 year] (Rhamnus frangula)   17%
- **Burdock mature seed** (Arctium lappa)   9%
- ★ **Stillingia root** (Stillingia sylvatica)   9%
- **Oregon Grape root** (Berberis aquifolium)   9%
- ★ **Phytolacca root** (Phytolacca americana)   9%
- **Prickly Ash bark** (Xanthoxylum clava-herculis)   9%
- ★ **Wild Indigo root** (Baptisia tinctoria)   4%
- **Potassium Iodide, USP**   (3% w/v)

★ Fresh   • Dried

ACTION
The Hoxsey Formula is a classic example of what the medical herbalist calls an "**alterative**" or "**depurative**," and in traditional folk medicine is known as a "**blood purifier**." It acts through the lymphatic, glandular and mucous membrane systems, and to a lesser degree through the skin. Its primary action is to favorably alter disordered processes of the metabolic & catabolic humors, especially those associated with the breakdown and elimination of metabolic waste. Its related secondary action is to enhance better overall absorption & assimilation of nutrients.

USES
Indicated in all constitutional disorders associated with tardy breakdown and elimination of metabolic & catabolic wastes, deterioration of normally healthy tissues, and slow reconstruction of new tissues (**retrograde metabolism, dyscrasia & cachexia**). Specific for **chronic congestion and swelling in the lymphatic & glandular systems**: lymph nodes, parotid, thyroid, thymus, pancreas, liver, spleen, Peyer's patches, prostate & ovaries. Also specific in chronic irritation & congestion of the mucous membranes (especially those of the bronchi, larynx, throat, & nasal cavities): **laryngitis**, **bronchitis**, **pharyngitis** & **sinusitis**. Can also be helpful in **chronic constipation**, **arthritis**, **skin diseases** (especially moist, red, irritable skin) & **chronic middle ear infections**. Also indicated as adjunct therapy in the treatment of **cancer**.

DOSE

Three times per day take 30 to 40 drops in a little water. Best taken between meals. While taking this compound drink plenty of water throughout the day.

Continued use in obstinate conditions: Take drops 2 times per day, 6 days per week, 3 weeks per month.

ADJUNCT THERAPY

To activate and potentiate the immune system add 30 to 40 drops of ECHINACEA EXTRACT to each dose of the above.

CAUTIONS

Do not take this compound if you are pregnant or nursing.

This compound is to be taken for chronic conditions only. It is not to be taken for acute conditions associated with fever, infection or inflammation.

With some individuals this compound can be laxative. This is not necessarily undesirable, but the dosage should be adjusted so its action is gentle and not severe. If gastric or intestinal discomfort occurs, use LAVENDER SPIRITS COMPOUND, or drink some hot tea made from any one or any combination of the following seeds: *fennel, anise, caraway, dill, or coriander.*

All of the health problems listed above can lead to serious medical consequences. If symptoms persist, and especially if there is fever, promptly seek qualified healthcare.

RUE • FENNEL COMPOUND
Herbal Eyewash

A blend of the liquid extracts of:
* ★ **Rue tops with immature fruit** (Ruta graveolens) 20%
* • **Fennel seed** (Foeniculum officinale) 20%
* ★ **Eyebright flowering herb** (Euphrasia officinalis) 20%
* • **Goldenseal rhizome & roots** (Hydrastis canadensis) 20%
* ★ **Mullein flower** [without stalk] (Verbascum thapsus) 20%

  Boric Acid, USP (1% w/v)

★ Fresh • Dried

ACTION & USES
A refreshing tonic for the eyes. Mildly soothing, cleansing and astringent. Especially indicated for "**tired eyes**" and for burning and inflamed eyes and conjunctiva: **allergies**, **conjunctivitis** ("pink-eye"), and "**bloodshot eyes**." Although not a specific for problems like failing vision, cataracts, glaucoma, or retinal displacement, this compound may nonetheless be indicated as adjunct therapy for enhancing overall ocular health.

DOSE
Never place undiluted drops directly in the eyes!
Place 3 to 15 drops* in an eyecup filled with *saline solution* and stir with the glass dropper until well mixed. Do an eyewash with this mixture (approximately 1 or 2 minutes for each eye) 1 to 3 times per day. While doing the wash make sure to keep the eye widely opened and rotate the eye in all directions.

* The number of drops that can be tolerated will vary with the individual and their situation. If the wash seems too strong, lower the number of drops until it feels comfortable.

* If eye is very irritated, inflamed, or infected start with 3 to 5 drops and add more drops only if they can be well tolerated.

Note: Take extreme care not to contaminate the dropper or the mouth of the bottle. Sterilize the eyecup before each use (boil for 5 minutes).

CAUTIONS
Discontinue use of this compound if it creates redness or irritation.

If symptoms of eye irritation, infection or injury are severe or persist for more than a few days, and especially if there is fever, promptly seek qualified healthcare.

ST. JOHN'S WORT • KAVA COMPOUND
Depression & Anxiety Remedy

A blend of the liquid extracts of:
★ **St. John's Wort flower & bud** (Hypericum perf.)   35%
● **Kava rhizome & roots** (Piper methysticum)   30%
★ **Skullcap flowering herb** (Scutellaria lateriflora)   25%
● **Prickly Ash bark** (Xanthoxylum clava-herculis)   10%
★ Fresh   ● Dried

ACTION & USES
Mild relaxing sedative, antispasmodic & muscle relaxant. This compound is indicated in **depression** & **despondency**, and associated **anxiety, nervous agitation, stress, restlessness** & **sleeplessness**.

While it can often help in relieving anxiety it can not be relied upon during panic attacks. However, its use over time may help to decrease the intensity and frequency of panic attacks.

For positive results in the treatment of depression its use must be continued for several weeks to several months. However, it should not be relied upon (esp. by itself) in the treatment of severe or manic depression, psychosis, or suicidal tendencies.

DOSE
Three to five times per day take 30 to 50 drops in water or chamomile tea.

ADJUNCTS
For adrenal support and to increase overall energy without using stimulants, take 30 to 40 drops of SIBERIAN GINSENG EXTRACT with each above dose.

For additional support of the nervous system take 30 to 40 drops of AVENA • SKULLCAP COMPOUND with each dose of the above.

For sleeplessness VALERIAN • PASSIONFLOWER COMPOUND can often be helpful.

CAUTIONS
Neurotic depression & prominent anxiety can be very serious mental health problems; especially if there are suicidal tendencies, or acute anger or rage. Seek help from a qualified mental healthcare professional if symptoms seem troublesome or out of control.

SAW PALMETTO • CLEAVERS COMPOUND
Prostate Gland Tonic

A blend of the liquid extracts of:
- **Saw Palmetto berry** (Serenoa serrulata)   25%
- ★ **Nettle root** (Urtica dioica)   20%
- ★ **Pipsissewa leaf** (Chimaphila umbellata)   20%
- **Cleavers herb** (Galium aparine)   20%
- ★ **Thuja leaf** (Thuja occidentalis)   15%

★ Fresh   • Dried

ACTION
The collective actions of the herbs in this compound are: to promote healthy circulation to & within the prostate and to drain away congested tissue fluids; to soothe burning & irritation of the prostate and the urinary tract; anti-inflammatory; mildly diuretic.

USES
Indicated in the treatment of prostate gland maladies (both acute & chronic): **infections** of the prostate, and **prostatitis** (inflammation of the prostate); difficulty in passing urine & **nocturnal dripping**; **prostatelcosis** (ulceration of the prostate). Especially indicated in **benign prostatic hypertrophy** (swollen prostate). Is also an excellent tonic for maintenance of a healthy prostate.

DOSE
Chronic: Two to three times per day take 30 to 40 drops in water. Take 6 days per week for 2 to 6 months, depending on results.

Acute: Three to five times per day take 30 to 40 drops in water or tea.*

Tonic: Two times per day take 30 to 40 drops in water. Take 6 days per week for 2 to 4 weeks. Do this 1 or 2 times per year.

* For optimal results take with URINARY TEA BLEND. This is especially recommended in acute & subacute inflammatory conditions, and in chronic conditions associated with burning or irritation.

ADJUNCT THERAPY
RED CLOVER • STILLINGIA COMPOUND is suggested in chronic (non-inflammatory) conditions of the prostate where there is congestion & swelling, sluggish lymphatics, and/or prostatorrhea (catarrhal discharge). Two to three times per day take 20 to 40 drops. For best results take drops one-half hour before or after SAW PALMETTO • CLEAVERS COMPOUND.

ECHINACEA EXTRACT is indicated in infection and inflammation of the prostate. Add 30 to 40 drops to each dose of SAW PALMETTO•CLEAVERS COMPOUND.

CAUTIONS

Prostate gland health problems should be treated under the supervision of a qualified healthcare practitioner. This is especially important in prostate conditions associated with pain, fever & abnormal discharge.

SPILANTHES • USNEA COMPOUND
Anti-Fungal Remedy

A blend of the liquid extracts of:
- **Usnea lichen** (Usnea barbata)   29%
- ★ **Spilanthes flowering herb & root** (Spilanthes oler.)   28%
- **Oregano leaf & flower** (Origanum spp.)   28%
- **Pau d'Arco inner bark** (Tabebuia impetiginosa)   14%

  Tea Tree leaf [essential oil] (Melaleuca alternifolia)   1%

★ Fresh   • Dried

USES
Indicated in the treatment of fungal infections of the mouth, stomach, intestines, anus, vagina, nose, ear, and skin, as well as systemic fungal infections. Specific for **candidiasis** (vaginal, intestinal & systemic), **apthea** (thrush) & **stomatitis**, **ringworm**, **athlete's foot**, **toenail** & **fingernail fungus**, etc.

DOSE
Internal: Three to five times per day take 30 to 40 drops in a little water. For optimal results, take 30 to 40 drops of ECHINACEA EXTRACT mixed with each dose.

Topical: Saturate a cotton ball with the compound and wet the affected area several times per day, or tape it to the area and leave on until dry. For optimal results, internal doses as described above are also suggested.

Vaginal Douche: Mix 2 to 3 teaspoons into 32 ounces of warm water and douche once each day for 5 days — then rest (no douche) for 2 days. If need be, this program can be continued for 3 weeks, then skip a week (no douches), and then repeat as before. If any irritation occurs, discontinue use, or lower strength of douche to tolerance.

CAUTIONS
In cases of high or persistent fever or other serious symptoms, or if the fungus seems to be spreading, promptly seek qualified healthcare.

THUJA • GOTU KOLA COMPOUND

Connective Tissue Tonic

A blend of the liquid extracts of:

★ **Gotu Kola herb & root** (Centella asiatica)   20%
● **Hawthorn berry, leaf & flower** (Crataegus oxy.)   20%
★ **Echinacea root** (Echinacea purpurea)   20%
★ **Horsetail herb** (Equisetum arvense)   20%
★ **Thuja leaf** (Thuja occidentalis)   20%

★ Fresh   ● Dried

ACTION

Studies have shown that *asiaticoside* (a naturally occurring terpenoid compound found in Gotu Kola plants) stimulates rapid and healthy growth of the reticuloendothelium. Oral doses of *asiaticoside* have been shown to strengthen the skin, stimulate growth of hair & nails, promote vascularization of connective tissue, and enhance local and general leukocytosis.*

Gotu Kola has been used in the folk medicine of Madagascar, Sri Lanka & India in the treatment of **leprosy**, **varicose ulcers**, **lupus** and certain obstinate **eczemas**.*

*Clinical Applications of Centella asiatica (L.) Urb. by Theodor Kartnig of Institut für Pharmakognosie, Universitat Graz, Graz, Austria.

USES

To be used in the establishment and maintenance of healthy connective tissue, and to facilitate its healthy regeneration in cases of injury or disease. Indicated in the healing of **skin lesions** (abrasions, cuts, burns & ulcerations) and as a tonic for minimizing the aging & wrinkling of skin; stomach, duodenal & intestinal **ulcers**; **varicose veins** & **hemorrhoids**; **scleroderma**; repair of eroded, **arthritic joints**.

DOSE

Tonic & Chronic: One to three times per day take 30 to 40 drops in a little water.

Acute: Three to five times per day take 30 to 40 drops in a little water.

Topical: Gently massage into the area to be treated until liquid is well absorbed. May sting if liquid comes into contact with broken skin, the eyes or mucous membranes.

CAUTIONS

The maladies listed above can be serious health threats, and some can be deadly if not treated properly. It is therefore important that these problems be treated by a qualified healthcare practitioner.

TRAUMA DROPS
COMPOUND
Anti-Trauma Remedy

A blend of the liquid extracts of:
- **Calendula flower** (Calendula officinalis)   40%
- **Arnica flower** (Arnica montana)   30%
- ★ **St. John's Wort flower & bud** (Hypericum perf.)   30%

★ Fresh   • Dried

USES
Specific for treating physical trauma: after injurious accidents (**falls, auto accidents, hard blows, sprains,** etc.), burns and before and after **surgery.** Indicated in: **heart strain**; **strokes**; **delerium tremens**; **strained muscles, tendons** & **ligaments**; **fractures** & **dislocations**; impaired nerve & spinal innervation and any associated loss of **sphincter control** (especially urinary **incontinence**); **postpartum pain** & **soreness** (especially after difficult labor). Also indicated in **emotional trauma**: sudden bad news, violence, terror, hysteria, etc.

DOSE
Acute: Mix 15 to 30 drops in water and take at once. Then take 5 to 10 drops every 1 to 2 hours as needed. Do not exceed 150 drops per day.
Caution: *Do not give liquids to anyone who is not fully conscious.*

Tonic: One to three times per day take 10 to 20 drops in water.

Topical: Apply full strength (undiluted) to thermal or sun burns, but only if skin is not broken.

ADJUNCT THERAPY
For strains and injuries this compound is best used with topical applications of TRAUMA OIL COMPOUND.

CAUTIONS
This compound is not a substitute for emergency medical care. Traumatic injuries should be cared for by a qualified healthcare practitioner.

TRAUMA OIL COMPOUND

Anti-Trauma Remedy

A blend of the olive oil extracts of:
- **Calendula flower** (Calendula officinalis)   40%
- **Arnica flower** (Arnica montana)   30%
- ★ **St. John's Wort flower & bud** (Hypericum perf.)   30%

★ Fresh   • Dried

USES
Indicated in injuries, **strains** and **inflammations** of muscles, ligaments, tendons and joints: **fractures** & **dislocations**, **sprains**, **bruises**, **contusions, arthritic joints** & **rheumatic pains**.

DOSE
Massage gently into traumatized area until well absorbed, and then cover. Can be used with hot-packs or ultrasound if they are not contraindicated.

ADJUNCT THERAPY
This compound is an excellent topical complement to TRAUMA DROPS COMPOUND.

CAUTIONS
Discontinue use of this compound if it creates irritation (this is rare).

This compound is not a substitute for emergency medical care. Traumatic injuries should be cared for by a qualified healthcare practitioner.

TURMERIC • CHAMOMILE COMPOUND
Anti-Inflammatory Remedy

A blend of the liquid extracts of:
- **Turmeric rhizome** (Curcuma longa) 18%
- ★ **Chamomile flower** (Matricaria chamomilla) 18%
- **Meadowsweet leaf & flower** (Spiræa ulmaria) 18%
- **Licorice root** (Glycyrrhiza glabra) 18%
- ★ **St. John's Wort flower & bud** (Hypericum perf.) 18%
- **Arnica flower** (Arnica montana) 10%

★ Fresh • Dried

ACTION
The predominant herbal constituents in this compound are flavonoids, salicylates ("herbal aspirin"), sesquiterpenes, and phytosterols ("herbal cortisone"). Through their antihistaminic, antioxidant, antipyretic (fever reducing), and vascular stabilizing actions these constituents help relieve the intensity and duration of the inflammatory process, minimize any associated tissue damage, and speed healing.

USES
This compound is not a remedy for any particular disease or injury, but instead is a specific for any associated inflammation. It is indicated in both **acute** & **chronic inflammations**, and it can be used as adjunct anti-inflammatory therapy in the treatment of: tissue injury or irritation, infections, fevers, allergies, mucous membrane inflammations (sinusitis, stomatitis, gastritis, colitis, etc.), hepatitis, nephritis, arthritis, dermatitis, phlebitis, tuberculosis, etc. May also be helpful in relieving inflammation associated with autoimmune diseases.

DOSE
Acute: Three to five times per day take 30 to 50 drops in a little water.* Best taken between meals.

Chronic: Three times per day take 30 to 40 drops in a little water.* Best taken between meals.

Topical application: Apply gently to inflamed area. Can be used undiluted in most cases but should be diluted (50 drops per ounce of water) for broken skin, ulcerations, sensitive areas and hemorrhoids.

ADJUNCT THERAPY

Use Echinacea Extract to potentiate a favorable immune response to inflammation. Take 30 to 40 drops with each dose of the above.

CAUTIONS

* For painfully inflamed stomach and intestines it is best to dilute drops in at least 8 to 12 ounces of water. If drops irritate the condition, discontinue their use.

Any inflammatory condition which is rapid in its onset, severe, painful, or persistent should be treated by a qualified healthcare practitioner.

URINARY TEA BLEND
Soothing Diuretic Tea

A blend of dried & cut herbs

Goldenrod flowering tips (Solidago canadensis)	25%
Marshmallow leaf (Althaea officinalis)	20%
Parsley leaf & root (Petroselinum hortense)	20%
Horsetail herb (Equisetum arvense)	20%
Black Elderberry (Sambucus nigra)	15%

ACTION & USES
A soothing **diuretic** that is both cleansing and tonic to the kidneys and bladder. It is especially indicated in **"scalding urine"** and other **irritations & inflammations of the urinary tract**. Helps remove excess water from the body by increasing urine output.

DOSE
To prepare tea: In the evening add 1 heaping tablespoon of tea blend to a quart jar, pour in 16 ounces of boiling water and stir well. Attach snug fitting lid to jar and let set overnight. In the morning strain tea well, using pressure to squeeze out as much tea as possible.

Drinking tea: Drink the above quantity of tea by *sipping* it throughout the day. For best results drink tea at room temperature (not hot).

ADJUNCT THERAPY
This tea is excellent when taken alone, but for optimal results (especially in infections) it is best taken with GOLDENROD•HORSETAIL COMPOUND.

CAUTIONS
Urinary infections can sometimes lead to serious medical consequences. If urinary symptoms persist for more than a few days, and especially if there is fever, promptly seek qualified healthcare.

VALERIAN • PASSIONFLOWER COMPOUND
Sedative Nervine & Sleep Tonic

A blend of the liquid extracts of:

★ **Valerian rhizome & roots** (Valeriana officinalis) 20%
★ **Passionflower flowering tips** (Passiflora inc. & edu.) 20%
• **Hops strobile with lupulin resin** (Humulus lupulus) 20%
★ **Chamomile flower** (Matricaria chamomilla) 20%
★ **Catnip leaf & flowering tips** (Nepeta cataria) 20%

★ Fresh   • Dried

ACTION
This compound is a gentle but effective **sedative** which is soothing and quieting to the nervous system. It is not narcotic, nor does it create any sense of being "drugged."

USES
Indicated in **nervous excitement** and **hysteria**, **mental depression** due to worry or imagined wrongs, **nervous headache**, and in nervousness associated with **menopause**. It is also specific for **insomnia**, as it allows the person to relax into a restful sleep and awaken fully refreshed.

DOSE
General Sedative: Two to five times per day take 30 to 40 drops in a little water.

Insomnia: Mix 15 to 30 drops in a little water and take 1 hour before bed and again just before bed. Usually works best after 2 to 4 nights of use.

CAUTIONS
Emotional and mental disease, and severe cases of mental depression should be treated by a qualified mental healthcare practitioner.

WILD CHERRY • PETASITES COMPOUND
Cough & Respiratory Congestion Remedy

A blend of the liquid extracts of:
- **Wild Cherry bark** (Prunus virginiana)   20%
- ★ **Petasites rhizome & roots** (Petasites officinalis)   20%
- **Skunk Cabbage rhizome & roots** (Dracontium fœtida)   20%
- **Licorice root** (Glycyrrhiza glabra)   20%
- **Thyme leaf & flower** (Thymus vulgaris)   20%

★ Fresh   • Dried

ACTION
Relieves coughs and irritation of the respiratory tract through the herbs' soothing, antispasmodic, anti-inflammatory and expectorant actions.

USES
Indicated in **coughs** associated with **respiratory congestion** of colds, flu, bronchitis and other pulmonary & bronchial affections.

DOSE
Adults: Two to five times per day take 20 to 40 drops in a little water.

Children: Two to five times per day take 5 to 15 drops in a little water.

To make a **cough syrup**, mix drops into a spoonful of honey, maple syrup or malt syrup.

ADJUNCT THERAPY
WILD CHERRY • PETASITES COMPOUND is a "general broad-specturm formula" designed to treat all types of coughs. However, the addition of certain other herbs to this compound can custom tailor it to fit a specific type of cough and thereby enhance the effectiveness of the treatment. If indicated, add one or two of the herbal extracts listed below to each dose of the compound:

SUNDEW EXTRACT (30 to 40 drops): dry, spasmodic or explosive coughs such as in whooping cough or measles; tickling coughs.

ELECAMPANE EXTRACT (30 to 40 drops): chronic coughs with persistent, teasing character and profuse expectoration; excellent for pulmonary infections.

YERBA SANTA EXTRACT (30 to 40 drops): chronic coughs with free secretions, especially in bronchitis & bronchorrhea.

GRINDELIA EXTRACT (30 to 40 drops): harsh, dry, unproductive coughs, especially with pectoral soreness or rawness; specific in subacute or chronic bronchitis, especially in the elderly.

BLOODROOT EXTRACT [1:10 strength] (15 to 20 drops): hacking coughs with loud mucous rales & difficulty in raising sputum; use only after active inflammation has subsided, and in atonic conditions. Always take Bloodroot extract well diluted with water. Lower dosage accordingly for small children (see Clark's Rule, pg. 128), and do not use Bloodroot during pregnancy.

CAUTIONS

Do not give this compound to children under 2 years of age unless directed by a physician. A persistent cough may be a sign of a serious condition. If cough or other symptoms persist for more than 7 days, tend to recur, or are accompanied by fever, rash, or persistent headache, promptly consult a qualified healthcare practitioner.

WILLOW • MEADOWSWEET COMPOUND

Analgesic (Pain Relieving) Remedy

A blend of the liquid extracts of:
- **Jamaican Dogwood root bark** (Piscidia erythrina) 25%
- ★ **Petasites rhizome & roots** (Petasites officinalis) 25%
- ★ **St. John's Wort flower & buds** (Hypericum perforatum) 20%
- ★ **Meadowsweet leaf & flower** (Spiræa ulmaria) 20%
- **Willow bark** (Salix lucida) 10%

★ Fresh   • Dried

ACTION

White Willow bark and Meadowsweet herb both contain the natural glycoside, *salicin,* which has a very similar chemistry to aspirin (acetylsalicylic acid). Salicin also has the same antipyretic (fever reducing), anti-inflammatory, and analgesic (pain relieving) properties as aspirin.

The word *aspirin* is derived from Meadowsweet's botanical name, *Spiræa.*

USES

This compound can give relief from many kinds of pain, and often is able to eliminate some pains completely. Indicated in **neuralgia**, **myalgia**, **enteralgia** & **visceralgia**, **headache**, **toothache**, **arthritis**, **lumbago**, **sciatica**, **painful spasms**, pain of **physical injuries**, painful **hemorrhoids**, **tic-douloureux**, **dysmenorrhœa** (painful menstruation), etc.

Although this compound often works well, nothing, beyond narcotics or anesthesia, can be expected to eliminate every kind and degree of pain.

DOSE

Adults: Three to five times per day take 30 to 40 drops in a little water.

Children: Adjust above adult doses according to child's body weight (see Clark's Rule, pg. 128).

Topical: Massage into painful area until well absorbed.

CAUTIONS

Pain can often be indicative of a more serious health problem. If pain persists, and especially if it is associated with fever, promptly seek qualified healthcare.

FREQUENTLY ASKED QUESTIONS ABOUT LIQUID HERBAL EXTRACTS

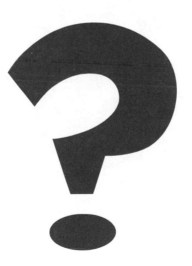

FREQUENTLY ASKED QUESTIONS
ABOUT LIQUID HERBAL EXTRACTS

What is a liquid herbal extract?

A liquid herbal extract is a concentrated liquid containing an herb's chemical constituents dissolved into a solution of alcohol and water. They are made by extracting ("washing") the herb's chemical constituents out of the inert herb fiber (cellulose) with a solution of alcohol and water. A good liquid herbal extract should optimally preserve the aroma, taste and biological activity of the herb from which it is made. Vanilla extract is a commonly known liquid herbal extract.

Are extracts made from fresh herbs better than ones made from dry herbs?

Many people assume that a fresh herb extract is superior to a dry herb extract, but this is not necessarily true; it really depends upon the unique biochemical, biophysical and energetic properties of the specific herb being extracted. While some herbs do indeed make a superior extract when extracted while still fresh and succulent (e.g., Shepherd's Purse, Corn Silk), there are also many herbs which make a superior extract when extracted after the herb is dried (e.g., Hops, Grindelia). Also, some herbs are best extracted when semi-dried (e.g., Saw Palmetto), or fermented (e.g., Wild Cherry, Sweet Clover), or some are toxic when fresh and must be dried and aged one year before they can be used safely (e.g., Buckthorn, Cascara Sagrada).

For thousands of years people have been successfully using hundreds of different herbs for healing, and while some are used fresh, the vast majority are used in their dry form. Remember that each herb has its own unique properties and therefore must be extracted accordingly. There are no universals when it comes to herbal extraction.

What is the purpose of alcohol in liquid herbal extracts?

The grain alcohol used to prepare liquid extracts serves three specific purposes. First, alcohol is the only edible solvent that will extract and preserve many of the naturally occurring herb constituents that are poorly soluble in water, such as essential oils, resins, balsams and many alkaloids. Second, alcohol is an excellent natural preservative, which maximizes the shelf-life of the extracts. Thirdly, alcohol is a great carrying agent which facilitates the absorption of the herb's constituents into the bloodstream.

Why is there so much alcohol in liquid herbal extracts and how much am I really taking?

The amount of alcohol in individual liquid extracts can vary from 20% to 90% depending on the herb being extracted and its content of alcohol and water soluble constituents. For example, to fully extract Cayenne's alcohol-soluble pungent resins and orange-red pigments requires at least 82% alcohol. A Cayenne extract made with a lower amount of alcohol will contain smaller amounts of Cayenne's resins and pigments, and therefore will be of lower quality than the higher alcohol extract.

The amount of alcohol you actually consume in a dose of liquid extract is actually very small. For example, taking 30 drops of Echinacea liquid extract (alcohol content of 45% to 50%) amounts to consuming 1/65th of a can of beer or 1/85th of an 8-ounce glass of wine. Also, if you mix those 30 drops of Echinacea liquid extract into 2 ounces of water, that mixture would contain only 0.59% alcohol.

Can I evaporate away the alcohol in liquid herbal extracts by mixing the extract drops into hot water?

A small amount of the alcohol can be removed this way but most of it will stay intimately mixed with the hot water and will remain so even if the water is boiled. That's because alcohol and water are chemical azeotropes and therefore are extremely difficult to separate once they have been mixed. While adding extracts to hot water will not eliminate their alcohol, it can, in some cases, actually damage the extract. Many extracts are heat stable (e.g., Goldenseal) and adding them to hot water does no harm. However, other extracts are damaged by heat (e.g., Valerian) and can be weakened by adding them to hot water. Also, essential oils and other non-water-soluble aromatic compounds found in certain extracts (e.g., Lemon Balm, Chamomile) do not mix well with water and can therefore evaporate away from the hot water. Here you are left with a compromised extract, but the alcohol remains.

How is the best way to take liquid herbal extracts?

Generally I prefer to mix the prescribed number of extract drops into 2 to 4 ounces of water. You can also add the drops to warm tea (not hot) or juice. Certain herbs, because of their stronger action, require more water and these have been so noted under "Dose" in this manual. For optimal results sip the mixed drops so you can savor the extract's flavor and aroma, although you may not always like the taste.

How many times per day should I take a dose of a liquid herbal extract?

Most of the doses in this manual recommend taking the extract "2 to 5 times per day." Normally 2 to 3 times per day is sufficient in chronic, ongoing conditions (e.g., poor memory, varicose veins). However, 4 to 5 times per day may be needed in acute, immediate conditions (e.g., fevers, colds). In a condition like chronic asthma, 2 to 3 times per day could be used on an ongoing basis, but could be increased to 4 to 5 times per day when there is an asthma flare-up.

What is the proper dosage of liquid herbal extracts for children?

Unless otherwise noted, all doses given in this manual are for adults, but Clark's Rule can be used to convert the adult dose to a child's dose.

> ## Clark's Rule
>
> Divide the child's weight (in pounds) by 150 to get the approximate fraction of the adult dose to give to the child.
>
> *Example:* For a 50 pound child give 50/150 (or 1/3) of the adult dose. Therefore, if the adult dose is 30 drops taken 3 times per day, the child's dose will be 10 drops taken 3 times per day (not 30 drops taken 1 time per day).

How many drops are in a one-ounce bottle of liquid herbal extract?

The number of drops in a bottle of liquid extract will vary depending on the viscosity (thickness) of the extract and its molecular weight. For example, one ounce of Herb Pharm's Goldenseal liquid extract contains 1,243 drops, Echinacea liquid extract contains 1,184 drops, and Comfrey liquid extract, which is very viscous, contains only 1,000 drops. In general, most extracts fall within the range of 1,000 to 1,300 drops per ounce.

How can I compare the dosage of herb capsules or tablets to the dosage of liquid herbal extracts?

Liquid herbal extracts are much easier to absorb and assimilate into the body than herb capsules and tablets. Herb capsules and tablets made from crude herb have to be digested (i.e., extracted) by the body before the herb's chemical constituents can be absorbed into the bloodstream. Since many herbs are very woody, digesting and absorbing them can be very difficult, especially for people with health problems. Therefore, much of the capsule or tablet remains undigested and never gets absorbed. However, the chemical constituents in a liquid herbal extract have already been "digested" and can therefore be readily absorbed into the bloodstream. Because of these differences, liquid herbal extracts are a much more efficient means of getting the chemical constituents out of the crude herb and into the bloodstream where they can do their healing work. Because of the widely varying amount of hard-to-digest woody fiber in various herbs and the efficiency of absorbing and assimilating liquid extracts, I always recommend using the dosage listed on the liquid extract's label or in this manual.

What is the meaning of "pyrrolizidine alkoloids removed" on your Comfrey, Coltsfoot and Petasites liquid extracts?

About 3% of flowering plants contain a group of chemical compounds called pyrrolizidine alkaloids (PAs); Comfrey, Coltsfoot and Petasites are in this group of plants. PAs can have a toxic effect on the liver when taken orally in large amounts or for extended periods of time. The amount of PAs in plants can vary greatly depending upon the botanical species and variety, growing conditions, plant part, and time of harvest. Occasional, small amounts of PAs are harmless to the body, but they can be cumulative. Children, the elderly and those with liver disease are more easily harmed by PAs and the fetus is particularly susceptible.

Because of safety concerns, Canada, Australia, England and several European countries have banned the sale of PA-containing herbs, although Germany and Switzerland do allow the sale of PA-free herbal products. The PAs can be removed by a chemical-free process (ion exchange) which removes nothing from the extract but the PAs and 2 to 3% of its minerals. The quality of these PA-free extracts is not compromised by this process and they can be used without concerns about PA toxicity. To assure safety, only use Comfrey, Coltsfoot or Petasites products that are free of PAs.

GLOSSARY

Acute condition - having a short and relatively severe course

Alterative - increases glandular activity and tissue metamorphosis

Analgesic - alleviates pain without causing loss of consciousness.

Antitussive - relieves or prevents coughs.

Antiphlogistic - counteracts inflammation, with fever.

Antipyretic - reduces the temperature of fevers.

Antispasmodic - prevents and relieves spasm of the voluntary and involuntary muscles.

Astringent - causes contraction of tissue and thereby restrains discharges.

Atonic - lacking normal tone or strength.

Bitters - group of herbs with bitter taste that increases the secretion of digestive juices.

Carminative - dispels accumulated gas in the stomach and bowels.

Catarrh - inflammation of a mucous membrane with increased flow of mucous.

Cholagogue - stimulates and increases the flow of bile.

Chronic condition - persisting over a long period of time.

Corrigent - favorably modifies the adverse effect or flavor of another herb.

Depurative - a purifying medicine.

Diaphoretic - promotes perspiration

Diuretic - causes and increases secretion and flow of urine.

Eliminant - promotes emptying of the bowel.

Emetic - causes vomiting.

Emollient - softens or soothes the skin, or soothes irritated mucosa.

Expectorant - facilitates the expulsion of sputum from the broncho-pulmonary mucosa.

Hemostatic - arrests the flow of blood.

Leukorrhea - a whitish, viscid discharge from the vagina and uterine cavity.

Modulator - regulates, adjusts or adapts.

Protective - affords defense against deleterious influences.

Resolvent - promotes softening and dissipation of inflammatory swelling.

Rubefacient - reddens the skin when applied topically.

Stomachic - promotes the functional activity of the stomach.

Stypic - arrests bleeding through a strongly astringent action.

Tonic - produces or restores normal tone to the functions and tissues of the body.

Vulnerary - promotes healing of wounds.

INDEX

Compounds are listed by page number.
Single herbs are listed by name.

Motion sickness 92, Basil, Ginger, Lavender

Mucous membranes 106, 116, Elecampane, Goldenseal, Myrrh, Nettle, Prickly Ash, Spilanthes, Stone Root

Mumps 96, Mullein, Red Root

Nausea 85, 92, Basil, Cardamon, Cramp Bark, Ginger, Lavender, Peppermint Spirits

Nephritis 82, 116, Gravel Root

Nervous system 61, 67, 105, 109, 119, Cactus, Celery, Chamomile, Hops, Kava, Lavender, Lemon Balm, Muira Puama, Oat Seed, Skullcap, St. John's Wort, Wild Yam

Pain 86, 87, 122, Arnica, Black Cohosh, Cal. Poppy, Meadowsweet, Petasites, St. John's Wort, Wild Yam

Phlebitis 68, Butcher's Broom

PMS 62, 85, 105, Black Cohosh, Butcher's Broom, Chaste Tree, Chamomile, Kava, Muira Puama

Poison oak, ivy, & sumac 84, Elder, Grindelia, Nettle

Postpartum 76, 85, 114, Black Cohosh, Cramp Bark, Wild Yam

Prenatal tonic 85

Prostate 106, 110, 118, Buchu, Cleavers, Gravel Root, Horsetail, Hydrangea, Meadowsweet, Nettle, Saw Palmetto

Psoriasis 64, Blue Flag, Burdock, Cleavers, Devil's Claw, Echinacea, Gotu Kola, Nettle, Prickly Ash

Puberty 85

Raynaud's Disease 80, Butcher's Broom, Ginkgo, Prickly Ash

Respiratory 74, 120, Coltsfoot, Comfrey, Elecampane, Goldenseal, Horehound, Mullein, Myrrh, Spilanthes, Usnea

Rheumatism 58, 94, 115, Angelica, Blue Flag, Cat's Claw, Celery, Devil's Claw, Devil's Club, Gravel Root, Juniper, Meadowsweet, Muira Puama, Prickly Ash

Ringworm 112, Bloodroot, Kava, Spilanthes, Usnea

Sciatica 122, St. John's Wort

Scleroderma 113, Gotu Kola

Seborrhea 64

Sedative 67, 119, Ashwagandha, Basil, Cal. Poppy, Catnip, Celery, Chamomile, Damiana, Hops, Kava, Lavender, Lemon Balm, Linden, Petasites, Skullcap, St. John's Wort, Violet

Sexual impotence 81, Cactus, Ginkgo, Chinese Ginseng, Muira Puama, Oat Seed, Yohimbe

Sexual tonic 81, Damiana, Ginkgo, Chinese Ginseng, Muira Puama, Oat Seed, Saw Palmetto, Yohimbe

Shingles 96, Cayenne, St. John's Wort

Sinusitis 77, 106, 116, Bayberry, Bloodroot, Coptis, Eyebright, Goldenseal, Usnea

Skin 106, 113, Burdock, Devil's Claw, Elder, Gotu Kola, Nettle, Violet

Sleep 109, 119, Cal. Poppy, Catnip, Chamomile, Hops, Kava, Lavender, Skullcap

Sore Throat 103, Arnica, Bayberry, Marshmallow, Mullein, Myrrh, Red Root, Usnea, Wild Indigo

Spasms 94, 122, Cramp Bark, Kava, Khella, Petasites, Wild Yam

Sprains 86, 114, 115, Comfrey

Steroids 89

Stomachache 101, Peppermint Spirits

Strained muscles & tendons 86, 114, 115, Arnica, Meadowsweet

Stress 61, 75, 109, Chinese Ginseng, Siberian Ginseng, Kava, Oat Seed

Stroke 83, 114, Arnica, Horse Chestnut

Surgery 114, Arnica, Butcher's Broom, Calendula, Stone Root

Swelling 94, Horse Chestnut, Mullein

Teething 67, Chamomile, Lemon Balm

Thyroid 63, Bladderwrack, Blue Flag, Bugleweed

Tic-douloureux 122, Kava

Tinnitus 99, Ginkgo

Tobacco addiction 60, Calamus

Toenail & fingernail fungus 112, Spilanthes

Tonsillitis 103

Toothache 122, Cal. Poppy, Feverfew, Kava, Meadowsweet

Trauma 87, 114, 115, Arnica, St. John's Wort

Ulcers 79, 113, Bayberry, Comfrey, Goldenseal, Gotu Kola, Licorice, Marshmallow, Myrrh, Wild Indigo, Yarrow

Urethritis 82, Buchu, Burdock, Gravel Root, Hydrangea, Kava, Saw Palmetto

Urinary tract 70, 82, 97, 118, Buchu, Celery, Cleavers, Corn Silk, Damiana, Goldenrod, Gravel Root, Horsetail, Hydrangea, Juniper, Kava, Marshmallow, Meadowsweet, Mullein, Saw Palmetto, Usnea

Urine, scalding 118, Cleavers, Goldenrod, Hydrangea, Marshmallow, Mullein, Violet

Urticaria 79, Nettle

Uterus 76, 85, Chaste Tree, Cramp Bark, Goldenseal, Gravel Root, Horse Chestnut, Saw Palmetto, Stone Root, Yarrow

Varicose veins 68, 80, 86, 113, Butcher's Broom, Calendula, Ginkgo, Gotu Kola, Hawthorn, Horse Chestnut, Milk Thistle, Stone Root, Yarrow

Veins 68, 80, Stone Root

Vertigo 93, 99, Ginkgo

Viral infections 96, Echinacea, Lemon Balm, Olive Leaf, St. John's Wort

Warts 96, Bloodroot

Whooping cough 94

NOTES